A short history of anaesthesia
The first 150 years

G. B. Rushman MB, BS, MRCS, LRCP, FRCA
Consultant Anaesthetist, Southend Hospital, Essex, UK

N. J. H. Davies MA, DM, MRCP, FRCA
Consultant Anaesthetist, Southampton General Hospital, Hants, UK

R. S. Atkinson OBE, MA, MB BChir, FRCA
Honorary Consulting Anaesthetist, Southend Hospital, Essex, UK

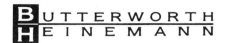

Butterworth-Heinemann
Linacre House, Jordan Hill, Oxford OX2 8DP
A division of Reed Educational and Professional Publishing Ltd

 A member of the Reed Elsevier plc group

OXFORD BOSTON JOHANNESBURG
MELBOURNE NEW DELHI SINGAPORE

First published 1996

British Library Cataloguing in Publication Data
A catalogue record for this book is available from the British Library.

Library of Congress Cataloguing in Publication Data
A catalogue record for this book is available from the Library of
Congress.

ISBN 0 7506 3066 3

Typeset by Interactive Sciences Ltd, Gloucester.
Printed and bound in Great Britain by Hartnolls Ltd Bodmin, Cornwall

Contents

Preface

The 1990s is a significant decade for anaesthetists: 1994, 1996 and 1997 are the 150th anniversaries of the first anaesthetics using nitrous oxide, ether and chloroform, respectively – the birth of modern anaesthesia. In addition, 1998 is the 100th anniversary of the first successful spinal anaesthetic.

There are relatively few great turning points in history. There can be no doubt, however, that the introduction of anaesthesia in the 1840s, followed in the 1870s by the introduction of antisepsis, was part of an explosion of new science and technology which was to alter for ever the direction of progress in medicine. It was a time of history in the grandest sense of that word. We have collected the main features of the exciting development of anaesthesia from the 1840s to the present day. The viewpoint is that of a British reader, but we are most conscious of the impact of discoveries made in other countries. We have not found room in this small volume for detailed description of apparatus, diagrams of which are already available elsewhere. We have referenced the text heavily, so that readers should be able to use this book as a springboard for research into most aspects of the history of anaesthesia.

Our aims have been, first, to document facts, with original sources; secondly to paint pictures of the pioneers of our subject; and thirdly to elucidate the undercurrents, significance and major changes of emphasis over the 150 years in question. Our subject cannot be confined to anaesthesia itself, and also must reach back before the 1840s to expose the foundations upon which these developments were based. The great pioneers of our speciality not only took the scientific lead, but their wisdom also secured the place which anaesthesia now holds in the world of medicine. This was not a result of chance. We have also included very recent history. In doing so, the selection of those aspects of present-day anaesthesia which will have an important impact on the future (without the benefit of the retrospectoscope!) has been challenging indeed.

Our sources have been the medical journals and proceedings of learned societies of the period. We are immensely grateful for four collections of historical material in London: the libraries of the Royal

Society of Medicine, Royal College of Surgeons, British Medical Association, and the Wellcome Institute for the History of Medicine. This book is essentially a book of facts. We are only too aware that there can be disagreement about such apparently simple things as dates of events. We have attempted to go back to original documents to verify these, but even then success is not always possible.

We owe an immense debt to Dr J. Alfred Lee, upon whose painstaking research and writing we have based our text. Much of his work was published in earlier editions of the *Synopsis of Anaesthesia*. We dedicate this volume to his memory.

G.B.R.
N.J.H.D.
R.S.A.

Acknowledgements

We are grateful for help and encouragement from Dr T. B. Boulton, Dr D. J. Wilkinson, Curator of the Charles King Collection, Dr I. McLelland, Librarian, Association of Anaesthetists of Great Britain and Ireland, Mrs J. Riordan, Archivist, Nuffield Department of Anaesthetics, Oxford, and to all our friends, who, over many years, have freely and enthusiastically shared their wisdom, insight and knowledge of historical matters. We are grateful for permission to reproduce the following illustrations: to the Wellcome Trust for Figures 1.1, 2.3, 16.1, to the Association of Anaesthetists of Great Britain and Ireland for Figures 2.1, 2.4, 2.5, 3.2, 4.2, 4.3, 4.4, 5.3, 7.2, 7.3, 7.4, 12.1, 15.4, 15.5, 18.1, 20.1, to the Royal College of Anaesthetists for Figure 1.3, to the Nuffield Department of Anaesthetics, Oxford, for Figures 5.4, 5.5, 18.2, to the late Dr J. A. Lee for Figures 1.2, 2.2, 3.1, 4.1, 4.5, 9.1, 13.2, 15.1, 15.2, 15.3, and to Dr D. J. Wilkinson for Figure 5.1.

1
The background to anaesthesia

Before the 1840s the mainstays of analgesia[1] during surgery were oral opium, laudanum (an opium derivative), mandragora (from the mandrake plant, *Mandragora officinarum*, a source of hyoscine and other alkaloids) and generous doses of alcohol. Psychological preparation was also important, and Anton Mesmer (1734–1815) introduced Europe to the supposed beneficial effects of 'mesmerism'. Literature is full of references to wondrous sleeping potions, ranging from Snow White's apple to Shakespeare (Cleopatra used mandrake). Yet the pioneering methods of producing satisfactory surgical anaesthesia were by inhalation of gases or vapours. Nitrous oxide was first used as a true anaesthetic in 1844, ether in 1846 and chloroform in 1847. It is not immediately apparent why drugs given by mouth should have been so completely supplanted by inhaled gases and vapours. In order to understand this, it is necessary to outline how the science of respiration developed over the preceding two centuries.

The discovery of the circulation of blood by William Harvey (1578–1657) led directly to the possibility of influencing any organ of the body by the single intravenous injection of a drug. His *Exercitatio Anatomica de Motu Cordis et Sanguinis in Animalibus* was published in 1628, although his experimental conclusions had been known several years before this. In 1665 Sir Christopher Wren (1633–1723) and Robert Boyle (1627–91) injected opium intravenously into a dog, and in the same year a German physician Johann Sigmund (1623–88) induced unconsciousness in the same way.

Oxygen and carbon dioxide

Harvey had observed the difference in colour between pulmonary arterial and venous blood, but he drew no firm conclusions about the function of the lungs. Between 1665 and 1675 Robert Hooke (1635–1703), Robert Boyle, Richard Lower (1631–91) and John

A short history of anaesthesia

Mayow of Oxford (1643–79) had gone a long way towards under-standing that a component of air was absorbed by the lungs, and that this process was necessary for both the life of a mouse and the burning of a candle.[2] The phlogiston theory of Joachim Becher and Georg Stahl then dominated thought in this field for nearly 100 years. Phlogiston was supposed to be a part of all combustible substances and to be liberated by their combustion and by an animal's respiration. When it accumulated in excess as a result of combustion or respiration in a closed container, it prevented further chemical activity. It was well known that some metals gained weight on combustion, and this meant that phlogiston had to have a negative weight. In brief, it was the very converse of oxygen.

Joseph Priestley (1733–1804) (Figure 1.1) prepared oxygen from saltpetre in 1771, as did Carl Wilhelm Scheele (1742–86). Priestley however is given the credit for discovering oxygen, or what he called 'dephlogisticated air', after liberating it in 1774 by heating red mercuric oxide using a focused magnifying glass.[3] He observed that this new gas was better than air at supporting respiration and combustion, but supposed this to be because it contained less phlogiston: 'dephlogisticated air'. It fell to Antoine Laurant Lav-oisier (1742–94) to clarify the use of oxygen in these processes and the simultaneous production of carbon dioxide (1777–78). He and the mathematician Pierre Simon Laplace[4] (1749–1827) coined the term 'oxygène' ('oxy' acid; 'gène' producer) in 1779, and were the first to compare the heat produced by respiration in animals with that from the combustion of carbon, and showed a relationship between oxygen used and carbon dioxide produced. Lavoisier was executed by the guillotine during the French Revolution. Justus von Liebig (1803–73), a Darmstadt chemist, showed in 1851 that carbo-hydrates and fats were substrates of metabolism, and not carbon itself.[5]

In the 1850s a French chemist, Boussingault, discovered that at a temperature of about 1000°C barium monoxide would absorb oxygen from air forming barium dioxide and release it at a higher temperature. This process was patented by his pupils the Brin brothers in the 1880s. Their company eventually became British Oxygen.

Carbon dioxide had been discovered by the Flemish chemist Jean Baptiste van Helmont (1577–1644) in the course of identifying many gases that were different to air. Van Helmont coined the word 'gas' derived from the Greek word *khos* = chaos. Carbon dioxide was isolated in 1757 by Joseph Black (1728–99), a Scottish chemist, who showed that it was produced not only by respiration and combus-tion, but also during fermentation. He named it 'fixed air'. Carbon dioxide was used to produce 'suspended animation' and surgical

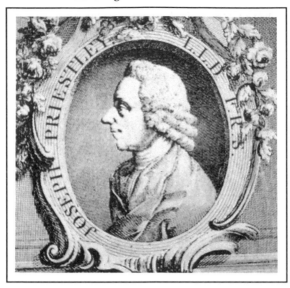

Figure 1.1   Joseph Priestley (1733–1804)[7]

Born in Fieldhead near Leeds, the son of a handloom worker, brought up in a strict nonconformist Calvinistic atmosphere by an aunt, and educated at Batley Grammar School. Trained as a dissenting minister and took charge of Mill Hill Chapel in Leeds in 1773. As a schoolmaster he experimented in chemistry, physics and electricity. Never stopped adhering to the phlogiston theory, unlike Lavoisier who discredited it. Spent seven years as librarian and companion to the second Earl of Shelbourne (1737–1805) at Bowood, Wilts.

Apart from preparing and identifying 'dephlogisticated air' (oxygen) in 1774, he also isolated or identified 'alkaline air' (ammonia), 'vitriolic acid air' (sulphur dioxide), 'dephlogisticated nitrous air' (nitrous oxide) in 1773 and 'nitrous acid air' (nitrogen dioxide). It is noteworthy that one of his teachers, Mathew Turner from Manchester, described the anaesthetic effects of ether in 1744.[8] Priestley also discovered methane, and the absorption of carbon dioxide by green plants in the presence of sunshine with the formation of oxygen. By subjecting carbon dioxide to pressure in water he discovered 'soda water'. Elected a Fellow of the Royal Society and he became a Doctor of Laws of the University of Edinburgh. From the former institution he received a Copley Medal for a paper[9] on 'The Different Kinds of Air'. His discoveries led Thomas Beddoes (1760–1808) of Bristol to experiment with the therapeutic effects of these various 'airs'.

In 1780 he went to Birmingham to take charge of a Unitarian congregation, The New Meeting House, and in this city he became a member of the famous Lunar Society which brought him into contact with Erasmus Darwin (1731–1802), physician and grandfather of Charles Darwin (1809–82), James Watt (1736–1818), scientist and inventor and William Murdoch (1757–1839), engineer and the inventor of gas lighting. Became a close friend of, and corresponded with, Benjamin Franklin (1706–90), the American printer, inventor and diplomat. An opponent of political discrimination against Dissenters, on the second anniversary of the fall of the Bastille (14 July 1789) his chapel, home, scientific apparatus, books and manuscripts were looted by a High Tory Royalist mob, forcing him to seek refuge in Hackney, near

London. His left-wing political opinions still separated him from his scientific colleagues, so that in 1794 he joined his sons in Northumberland, Pennsylvania. Here, he added farming to his other activities and soon became a leader of his new community. Died of oesophageal obstruction in 1804 at the age of 70. A statue of him was unveiled in Birmingham by Thomas Henry Huxley in 1874 to mark the centenary of the discovery of oxygen. Hilaire Belloc (1870–1953), the poet, journalist and historian, was a great-grandson.

anaesthesia in animals in 1824 by Henry Hill Hickman[6] (1800–30), described later.

The pneumatic treatment of disease

Just as Harvey's understanding of the circulation of blood had allowed the development of intravenous therapy, this basic scientific work on respiration led to the possibility of breathing gases and vapours for similar therapeutic reasons. Priestley himself experimented with various gases, especially while in Birmingham. One of his circle, Richard Pearson, recommended the inhalation of ether for lung diseases.

Thomas Beddoes (1760–1808), a physician and chemist at Oxford who was friendly with the group at Birmingham, founded an Institution at Clifton in Bristol for the study of such pneumatic therapy. He was helped by James Watt (1736–1819), the engineer, and received a large donation from Josiah Wedgwood. Among the gases that Beddoes recommended for patients were oxygen (used by him in medical treatment in 1794), carbon dioxide, 'water gas' (hydrogen, carbon monoxide and carbon dioxide), and hydrogen. The first use of oxygen in medicine was probably by Chaussier in 1780, including for neonatal asphyxia.[10]

In 1798 Beddoes met Humphry Davy (1778–1829) (Figure 1.2) while on holiday in Cornwall, and invited Davy (while still only 19 years old) to be the Superintendent of the Pneumatic Institution in Bristol. Here he undertook a series of experiments on the effects of breathing nitrous oxide. He described his personal observation of its analgesic effect[11] after he had acquired inflammation of the gums: 'On the day when the inflammation was most troublesome, I breathed three large doses of nitrous oxide. The pain always diminished after the first four or five respirations.' He went on to suggest that as it 'appears capable of destroying physical pain, it may probably be used with advantage during surgical operations in which no great effusion of blood takes place'.[12] This was the first suggestion that surgical analgesia might be achieved by inhalation. He also realized that pulmonary blood flow and hence cardiac output could be measured by estimating the rate at which nitrous

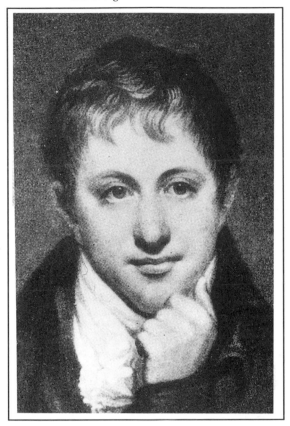

Figure 1.2 Humphry Davy (1778–1829)[14]

Born in Cornwall, the son of a wood carver. Became apprenticed to J. B. Borlase, surgeon, of Penzance, in 1795. At the age of 17 he had prepared nitrous oxide and examined the effects of its inhalation. In 1798 Davy became Superintendent of Thomas Beddoes's (1760–1808) Pneumatic Institution in Clifton, Bristol, for the treatment of pulmonary tuberculosis by inhalation of gases. Published the results of his work there in a book *Researches, Chemical and Philosophical; Chiefly Concerning Nitrous Oxide* (London: J. Johnson, 1800). In later life, Davy became famous. Moved from Bristol to direct the chemical laboratory at the Royal Institution, invented the miner's safety lamp, was created a baronet in 1818, and was elected President of the Royal Society in 1820. Among Davy's colleagues at Bristol was Dr Peter Mark Roget, FRS, famed for his *Thesaurus of English Words and Phrases* (1852). Davy prepared nitrous oxide by the method of Berthollet (1785) by heating ammonium nitrate. Taught Michael Faraday (1791–1867), and was the first to describe sodium and potassium.

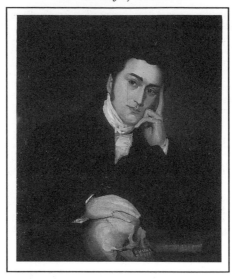

Figure 1.3   Henry Hill Hickman (1800–30)[14]

Born 27 January at Lady Halton, Bromfield, near Ludlow in Shropshire. Matriculated at Edinburgh University in November 1819 and was admitted as a Member of the Royal College of Surgeons of England on 5 May 1820. In 1821 he married Eliza Hannah Gardner and set up practice in Ludlow, probably at 114, Corve Street. On 21 February he wrote a letter to T. A. Knight, Esq. of Downton Castle stating that in his surgical practice he lamented the pain felt by many patients and claimed to have performed experiments on animals under the influence of carbonic acid gas without pain and with full recovery. Excised the ears, tail and legs of dogs and rabbits. His results were published in a paper, 'A Letter on Suspended Animation, Containing Experiments Showing that it may be Safely Employed during Operations on Animals, with the View of Ascertaining its Probable Utility in Surgical Operations on the Human Subject' (Ironbridge, 1824).[15] William Morton was only a child of 5 at this time. Even Sir Humphry Davy, who was approached directly by Knight, showed no interest.[15] Knight's main scientific interest was botany. In May 1824 the contents of his house in Ludlow were put up for sale, including a collection of stuffed birds and animals, and Hickman moved to Church Street in Shifnal, Shropshire. There he had printed as a pamphlet a fresh version of his letter to T. A. Knight, the greater part of which was reproduced in the Shrewsbury Chronicle in 1825. His work, however, attracted no attention from scientific men in Britain and in 1828 he visited Paris to present a memorial 'To his Most Christian Majesty Charles X of France'. This memorial was forwarded to the Académie Royale de Médecine and a committee set up to consider the matter. Only Baron Dominique Jean Larrey (1766–1842) showed any interest. Hickman returned to England a disappointed man, setting up practice in Teme Street in Tenbury Wells, Worcestershire. His house is now a restaurant. However he died within the year (1830), the cause of death not being known. Buried in the churchyard of St. Mary the Virgin, Bromfield, the church in which he had been baptised.

The first allusion to Hickman in recent times was made in an article by Thompson[6] in 1912. In 1930 the Section of Anaesthetics of the Royal Society of Medicine erected a memorial in the church which was unveiled by Sir St. Clair Thompson and dedicated by the Bishop of Hereford.[16] The Wellcome Historical Medical Museum in London was responsible for a Centenary Exhibition in 1930. The Section of Anaesthetics of the Royal Society of Medicine now awards a Hickman Medal to a distinguished recipient every three years. The Royal College of Anaesthetists possesses a chest which had belonged to Hickman. Other possessions of Hickman include an inkwell in the Ludlow Museum and an original miniature of Eliza Hickman in the museum in Tenbury Wells.

---

oxide is taken up by the lungs. A nitrous oxide container was made by James Watt in 1799 to assist this research.[13]

The idea of deliberately inhaling nitrous oxide to produce surgical analgesia was not pursued by Humphry Davy or anyone else at this stage. However his work was known to, and may have influenced, Gardner Quincy Colton (1814–98) 44 years later. Curiously, gases and vapours were not inhaled only in the hope that they might help various diseases, but also for pure entertainment and amusement. Davy named nitrous oxide 'laughing gas'. This form of entertainment seemed to be without any long-term harm, and was widespread in certain social circles. The poets Robert Southey and Samuel Taylor Coleridge both described the effects of nitrous oxide given by Davy. A similar use of ether vapour ('ether frolics') was exploited in America.

The first deliberate use of an inhaled gas to produce anaesthesia for the performance of surgical operations in animals was carried out by Henry Hill Hickman (Figure 1.3) in 1823 and 1824 using carbonic acid gas (carbon dioxide), but this contribution was not recognized by medical opinion at that time.

References

1. The history of pain relief for surgery before the 1840s is described by a series of papers in *A History of Anaesthesia*, edited by R. S. Atkinson and T. B. Boulton, Royal Society of Medicine, London, 1989. There is an excellent survey of this period by Boulton, T. B. and Wilkinson, D.J. 'The origins of modern anaesthesia,' in *A Practice of Anaesthesia*, 6th edn, edited by T. E. J. Healy and P. J. Cohen, Edward Arnold, London, 1995.
2. Mayow, J. *Tractactus Quinque Medicophysici*, No.2. Oxford, 1674.
3. Priestley, J. *Phil. Trans.*, 1772, **52**, 147; *Experiments and Observations on Different Kinds of Air*, 1774, vol.1; (1775), vol.2, sect.III–V, pp.29–103 (reprinted in 'Classical File', *Surv. Anesthesiol.*, 1976, **20**, 81)
4. Lavoisier, A-L. and Laplace, P. S. *Mém. Prés. Acad. Sci. Paris*, 1780, **103**, 566
5. Liebig, J. *Letters on Chemistry*, 3rd edn, 1851
6. Thompson, C. J. S. *Br. Med. J.*, 1912, **1**, 843

7. See also Smith W. D. A. *Under the Influence: A History of Nitrous Oxide and Oxygen Anaesthesia*, Macmillan, London, 1982; and McDowell, D. G. *Anaesth. Intensive Care*, 1982, **10**, 4
8. Fuller, J.F. *Anesthesiology*, 1947, **8**, 464
9. 'Classical File', *Surv. Anesthesiol.*, 1976, **20**, 283
10. Hahn, L. L'oxygène et son emploi médical. *Janus*, 1899, **4**, 6
11. Excerpts reprinted in *Surv. Anesthesiol.*, 1968, **12**, 92;
12. Davy, H. *Researches, Chemical and Philosophical; Chiefly Concerning Nitrous Oxide*, J. Johnson, London, 1800; also facsimile reproduction, Butterworths, London, 1972
13. Cartwright, F. F. *Proc. 4th World Cong. Anaesth.*, 1968, 203
14. See also Cartwright, F. F. (1952) *The English Pioneers of Anaesthesia*, Wright, Bristol; and Bryn-Thomas, K. *Anaesthesia*, 1978, **33**, 903
15. Reprinted in 'Classical File', *Surv. Anesthesiol.*, 1966, **10**, 92
16. Reception at Wellcome Historical Museum, *Br. Med. J.*, 1930, **1**, 713–714

2
The first two years of anaesthesia

By the 1840s the inhalation of gases and vapours for sheer fun was common on both sides of the Atlantic. Although Hickman had been the only person to suggest that such a technique could be deliberately used to produce anaesthesia for surgical operations, and moreover had demonstrated its success in animals, he was unfortunate to have chosen carbon dioxide. It was only a matter of time before a more useful agent was chosen. Nitrous oxide and ether were separately introduced within a few years of each other, and their use was pivotal in the origins of inhalational anaesthesia as we know it today. Nitrous oxide is of course still in daily use throughout the world. By contrast ether, which rapidly became the main anaesthetic for over a century, has given place to all the modern volatile agents, but is itself still an important agent in several continents.

Nitrous oxide

Joseph Priestley had first prepared nitrous oxide in 1772. He called it 'dephlogisticated nitrous air'. Sir Humphry Davy had suggested that its analgesic properties might be of value in surgery as early as 1800, but had taken the matter no further. The consequences of breathing 'laughing gas' were well known both to visitors at the Pneumatic Institution in Bristol and in America. P. C. Barton (1786–1828), of Philadelphia, described its exhilarating effects in 1808. Both he and the distinguished surgeon Willard Parker (1800–84) from New York may have influenced a peripatetic lecturer in chemistry, Gardner Quincy Colton (1814–98).

Gardner Colton (Figure 2.1) made a living by travelling up and down America giving popular scientific lectures. He often demonstrated the effects of nitrous oxide, and it is not difficult to imagine the appeal this would have to an audience. Although he had studied medicine, he never took his degree.

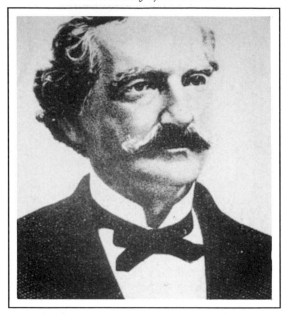

Figure 2.1   Gardner Colton (1814–98)

On the evening of 10 December 1844 Colton[1] gave his accustomed demonstration of the effects of inhaling nitrous oxide at Hartford, Connecticut. Horace Wells (1815–48) (Figure 2.2), a local dentist, was present. The demonstration was repeated privately the next day. Wells noticed that a young druggist's shop assistant, Samuel Cooley, while under the influence of the gas, banged his shin and made it bleed, but stated afterwards that he experienced no pain. Wells commented that nitrous oxide might therefore enable a tooth to be extracted painlessly. As it happened, his own wisdom tooth was causing him trouble, and he persuaded Colton to go to his surgery and try the gas on himself. The experiment was carried out that day (11 December 1844), with Colton as the anaesthetist and John M. Riggs (1810–85) as the dentist. It was a big success. When Wells recovered from the effects of the anaesthetic he famously proclaimed: 'a new era in tooth-pulling!' Wells learnt from Colton the method of manufacture of nitrous oxide and used it in his dental practice (assisted by Riggs) on 15 patients over the next month. It was administered from an animal bladder through a wooden tube into the mouth, while the nostrils were compressed.

Later Wells went to Boston, then the focus of medicine in northeastern America, to interest a larger audience in his discovery.

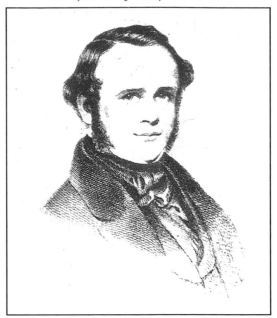

Figure 2.2 Horace Wells (1815–48)

Born in Hartford, Connecticut. Set up in dental practice in Hartford, and among his pupils was William Morton. Morton was Wells's partner in 1842–43, but the partnership was not successful. In 1847 Wells published[2] his letter: 'A History of the Discovery of the Application of Nitrous Oxide Gas, Ether, and Other Vapours to Surgical Operations'. In the same year he opened a dental office in New York City but soon afterwards gave up dentistry, became a chloroform addict, and travelled around the country with a troop of performing canaries. He was incarcerated in jail after bespattering a New York prostitute with sulphuric acid, while recovering from self-administered chloroform.[3] He commited suicide a few days later at the age of 33 by cutting his femoral artery.

William Morton had formerly been a partner in dental practice with Wells, and was able to introduce him to some of the surgeons at Massachusetts General Hospital, particularly Dr John Collins Warren (1778–1856). Wells was invited to demonstrate the use of nitrous oxide in 1845, on a patient having a dental extraction, to Warren's students at Harvard Medical School. The patient was too lightly anaesthetized and complained of pain. The affair was a fiasco and Wells was hissed out of the room as a fraud. William Morton and also Charles T. Jackson (1805–80) were present at this operation. Wells returned to Hartford and continued to use the gas, but the introduction of ether gradually ousted nitrous oxide, and the latter was temporarily forgotten. It was eventually reintroduced by Gardner Colton, again for dentistry, in 1863 in New Haven, Connecticut.

Ether

Before Morton's demonstration in October 1846

Diethyl ether was first prepared in 1540 by Valerius Cordus (1515–44), who called it sweet oil of vitriol. Sigmund August Frobenius, the German chemist, physician and botanist from Wittenberg, named it ether.[4] Together with nitrous oxide it had been used as a drug of amusement in both America and Europe.

An article by Walter Channing[5] suggested that the analgesic effects of ether were accidentally used in 1833 by an unknown chemist who wiped ether freely over the face of his wife during her prolonged labour and observed that her distress passed away. Channing also published 'A Treatise on Etherization in Childbirth illustrated by 581 Cases'.[6] Ether was probably first used for clinical anaesthesia by William E. Clarke (1819–98) of Rochester, New York, in January 1842, when the dentist Elijah Pope extracted a tooth from a Miss Hobbie.[7] This was not published at the time and did not attract attention.

Crawford Williamson Long (1815–78) (Figure 2.3), a general practitioner in Jefferson, Georgia had frequently inhaled ether. Just as Wells had observed in the case of nitrous oxide, Long noted that he could acquire painful knocks and bruises on his body while under the influence of ether without remembering the trauma. He too realized that this effect would be 'applicable in surgical operations'. He tried out this possibility on a patient of his, a young man called James M. Venable, on 30 March 1842.[8] Long excised one of two cysts on the back of his patient's neck, after administering ether from a towel. He continued to use ether over the next few years for minor surgery, but did not publish his results until later.[9]

Morton's demonstration of October 1846

The main credit for the introduction of ether as an anaesthetic agent belongs to William Thomas Green Morton (1819–68) (Figure 2.4). By the time that Long reported his work in 1849, Morton's fame was well established. In science, the recognition for a new discovery belongs to the man who convinces the world, not to the man to whom the idea first occurs. Morton convinced the world of the advantages of ether anaesthesia and so takes the laurels.

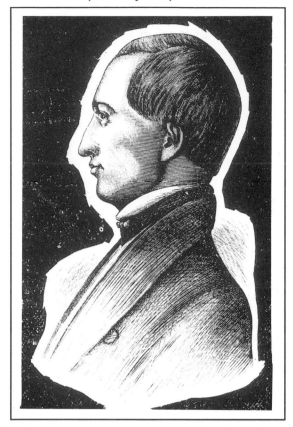

Figure 2.3   Crawford Williamson Long (1815–78)[10]

Born in Danielsville, Georgia, 1 February 1815, the son of a state senator. Graduated from the University of Pennsylvania in 1839 and after working in New York settled in general practice with his former tutor, Dr Grant, in Jefferson. A museum built on the site of Long's original surgery was dedicated in 1957, in Jefferson, Georgia.

Morton had moved from Hartford to Boston in 1843, and had set up his dental practice there. His speciality was prosthetic work, and so he was obliged to perform many dental extractions. He therefore had a direct humanitarian and financial interest in alleviating pain during these procedures. He had observed Wells's failure with nitrous oxide at the Massachusetts General Hospital in 1845. Ether was an obvious alternative, especially since he had observed its effects on his patients when they breathed the vapour after applying liquid ether to deaden painful tooth sockets. This had been the

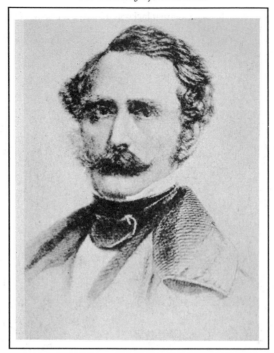

Figure 2.4   William Thomas Green Morton (1819–68)

Born in Charlton, Worcester County, Massachusetts, and started work at the age of 16 in a printing house. Later went into business, but this was a failure. As a young man he suffered the pain of a surgical operation, in Cincinnati. He studied at the Baltimore College of Dental Surgery, set up in practice at Farmington, Connecticut, and later became a pupil and then (1842–43) a partner of Horace Wells at Hartford. Separated from Wells and, becoming a medical student in Boston at the Harvard Medical School (1844), was present when Wells failed to satisfy the audience as to the efficiency of nitrous oxide. Never qualified in medicine, but received an honorary MD in 1852: 'This priceless gift to humanity went forth from the operating theatre of the Massachusetts General Hospital, and the man to whom the world owes it is Dr W. T. G. Morton.' The last 20 years of Morton's life was dominated by much wrangling between him and Charles T. Jackson (1805–80) as to whom should be given credit for the discovery. Morton also spent much time and effort attempting to patent ether under the name Letheon. One of the reasons for this effort was that he recognized the dangers of the administration of ether, but it became apparent that such a patent was not enforceable.[14] Morton three times petitioned the US Congress, and even obtained an interview with the President (Franklin Pierce, 1804–69), but he was never in his lifetime officially recognized as the pioneer of ether anaesthesia. Time later vindicated his claim, and Jackson revealed as someone trying to take the credit for someone else's work, as he had tried to do in other scientific arenas. Jackson became severely mentally ill in 1873, and died in 1880 in an asylum. Morton spent his later years farming at Needham, Massachusetts, and died of cerebral haemorrhage quite suddenly in Central Park, New York City, on 15 July 1868.[15] At the time of his death he was planning to file a lawsuit against Jackson. He died a disappointed man.[16] The inscription on his tombstone in Mount Auburn Cemetery, Boston, composed by Henry J. Bigelow, reads: 'Inventor and Revealer of Inhalation Anesthesia: Before Whom, in All Time, Surgery was Agony; By Whom, Pain in Surgery was Averted and Annulled; Since Whom, Science has Control of Pain.'

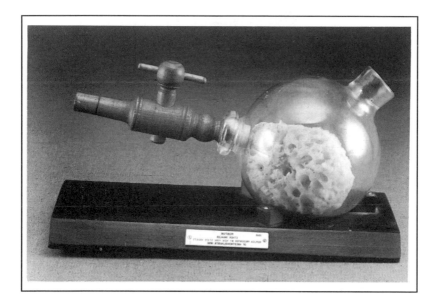

Figure 2.5   Morton's inhaler

suggestion of Charles T. Jackson (1805–80), a chemist and geologist who had taught Morton earlier in Boston.[11] Morton subsequently tried ether on himself, a dog, and his two young assistants, and although these were successful experiments, he felt he needed further chemical advice. He turned to Jackson, and this interaction laid the foundation for the later dispute between the two men as to who deserved the credit for the introduction of ether.

On 30 September 1846 a patient, Eben H. Frost, came to the surgery and was willing to breathe ether for a dental extraction.[28] The patient said that he 'did not experience the slightest pain whatever'. Morton gained further experience, including the administration of 37 anaesthetics for the surgeon Henry Jacob Bigelow (1818–90), surgeon and Professor of Materia Medica.

Morton, who throughout this time was most secretive about his techniques, then approached John Warren, the senior surgeon at Massachusetts General Hospital, to ask for the opportunity to make a public demonstration. This was arranged for just two days later, on 16 October 1846.[28] Morton made last-minute improvements to the glass flask that he used to administer the ether (Figure 2.5), including the addition of inspiratory and expiratory valves.

The operation was for the removal of a vascular tumour from just below the mandible, and took place in what is now the 'Ether Dome' at Massachusetts General Hospital. The patient (who gave 'informed consent') was a young man, Edward Gilbert Abbott (1825–55), a printer and journalist, and Warren was the surgeon.[12] Its success prompted Warren to remark to the audience around him at the completion of surgery: 'Gentlemen, this is no humbug.' After the operation the patient remained in hospital for 7 weeks.[13]

News of anaesthesia spreads

The news of Morton's discovery soon spread throughout the civilized world. In December 1846 Francis Boott (1792–1863), a physician born and trained in the USA but practising in Gower Street, London,[17] received news of pain-free surgery during the inhalation of ether. The news was conveyed in a letter that was written on 28 November by Jacob Bigelow (1786–1865), who was a friend of Boott and was Henry Bigelow's father. The letter had thus taken some three weeks to reach Boott. On 19 December 1846 Boott encouraged Mr James Robinson (1813–62)*, a dentist, to give ether to a Miss Lonsdale for the extraction of a molar, Robinson acting as dentist and anaesthetist.[21] This took place at Boott's study in Gower Street. The site is commemorated by a plaque.[22] Boott and Robinson

---

* James Robinson (1813–62)[18]

Born in Southampton of a naval family. Studied in Guy's Hospital and London University before setting up his dental practice at 7 (now 14) Gower Street. Had already become known for his attempts to set up dental organizations and for the foundation of a journal, *The Forceps* (which was to last only 15 months), before he was approached by his neighbour, Boott, to administer ether to Miss Lonsdale for the extraction of a molar tooth. The success of this first ether administration in England made him the most experienced administrator of ether than any other for a period of about 4 months.[19] Demonstrated his art to others: 'I again operated this morning with the most perfect success, in the presence of my friends – Mr Stocks, Mr Snow and Mr Fenney.'[20] Robinson became the author of the world's first textbook of anaesthesia: *A Treatise of the Inhalation of the Vapour of Ether* (Webster, London, 1847). In 1856 Robinson was a founder member and became first President of the short-lived College of Dentists, incorporated in the College of Surgeons in 1859, which in turn was involved in the foundation of the National Dental Hospital in 1861. In 1848, Robinson was appointed Surgeon Dentist to the Royal Free Hospital and, in 1949, Surgeon Dentist to H.R.H. Prince Albert. He died in Kenton, Middlesex in March 1862, at the early age of 48, following an accidental slippage of a knife in his garden which severed the femoral artery.

had arranged for Hooper of Pall Mall to construct an inhaler especially for this occasion. The pain-free extraction was reported later in the *Illustrated London News* on 9 January 1847.

So successful was the operation that Boott persuaded Robert Liston (1794–1847), Professor of Surgery at the University of London, to experiment with the new drug. It was tried out with considerable publicity and brilliant success for the amputation through the thigh of Frederick Churchill's leg at University College Hospital on 21 December 1846. Churchill was a 36–year-old butler.[23] Liston died of a ruptured aortic aneurysm a year after this operation. The apparatus used in this operation was designed by Peter Squire, the Queen's chemist and druggist (who in 1804 founded the *Companion to the British Pharmacopoeia*, which later became *Martindale's Extra Pharmacopoeia*), and was a modification of Dr Nooth's apparatus for the production of soda water. The ether was actually administered by the designer's nephew, William Squire, a medical student of 21[24]. When the leg had been painlessly amputated Liston said to the large audience: 'This Yankee dodge beats mesmerism hollow.'

Liston followed this operation with a second case, an avulsion of a toenail, which was equally successful. Joseph Lister (1827–1912), the pioneer of antisepsis and subsequently Professor of Surgery at the University of Glasgow, was working at University College Hospital in 1846, and was among the distinguished visitors present that day. Another doctor who may have been present, but less distinguished at that time, was Joseph Thomas Clover (1825–82), who was later to become such a prominent anaesthetist.

Ether was probably given in Scotland on 19 December (the same day as the dental extraction by Robinson in London) in the Dumfries and Galloway Royal Infirmary by William Scott (1820–87), surgeon, and William Fraser (1819–63), ship's surgeon, who had trained in Liverpool where his father was a local apothecary.[25] This followed a verbal report of Morton's successful use of the agent, carried by Fraser, who arrived in Liverpool from Boston on 16 December, as medical officer on the steamship *Acadia*. In Ireland the first anaesthetic was given by John MacDonnell in Dublin at the Richmond Hospital.

News spread quickly to all parts of the civilized world. Joseph François Malgaigne used ether in Paris, and reported his first five cases to the Académie de Médecine on 12 January 1847. He used apparatus designed to deliver the vapour nasally. The surgical instrument manufacturer in Paris, Charrière, constructed a flask in January 1847 that became popular for the administration of ether. Nikolai Ivanovitch Pirogoff (1810–81), a Russian military surgeon in

St. Petersburg, was successful in giving ether rectally.[26] He also administered ether intravenously to animals.

The name 'anaesthesia' was suggested by Oliver Wendell Holmes (1809–94), Professor of Anatomy and Physiology at Harvard Medical School, in a letter of 21 November 1846 to Morton. He wrote: 'Dear Sir, Everyone wants to have a hand in a great discovery. All I will do is to give you a hint or two as to names. . . . The state should, I think, be called "Anaesthesia". This signifies insensibility, more particularly (as used by Linnaeus and Cullen) to objects of touch. . . . The adjective will be "Anaesthetic". . . . I would have a name pretty soon . . . the terms, which will be repeated by the tongue of every civilised race of mankind. . . . You could mention these words which I suggest for their consideration.' The word anaesthesia had also appeared in Bailey's *English Dictionary* in 1721. It denoted loss of sensation, but not of consciousness.[27] Despite the subsequent adoption of the word anaesthesia, 'etherization' was widely used in the initial years.

References

1. Smith, G.B. and Hirsch, N.P. *Anesth. Analg.*, 1991, **67**, 185–193.
2. Published in Hartford, Conn., 1847 (reprinted in 'Classical File', *Surv. Anesthesiol.*, 1958, **2**, 1)
3. *Boston Med. Surg. J.*, 1848, **38**, 25
4. Frobenius, J.A.S. *Phil. Trans. R. Soc. Lond.*, 1729, **36**, 283; Bergman, N.A. *Proc. 3rd Internat. Symp. Hist. Anaesth.*, edited by B.R. Fink, L.E. Morris and C.R. Stephen, Wood Library-Museum of Anesthesiology, Park Ridge, Ill., 1992, pp.53–59
5. Channing, W. *Boston Med. Surg. J.*, 1852, **46**, 113–115
6. Channing, W. *A treatise on etherization in childbirth illustrated by 581 cases*, William D. Tichner and Co., Boston, 1848, 25pp.
7. Bigelow, H. J. *Am. J. Med. Sci.*, 1876, **141**, 164
8. Jeffereys, J. *Lancet*, 1872, **2**, 241; *Br. Med. J.*, 1872, **2**, 499
9. Long, C.W. *Sth Med. J.*, 1849, **5**, 705 (reprinted in 'Classical File', *Surv. Anesthesiol.*, 1960, **4**, 120); *J.A.M.A.*, 1965, **194**, 1008; Cole, W.H.J. *Anaesth. Intensive Care*, 1974, **2**, 92; Taylor F. *C.W. Long and the Discovery of Ether*, Hoebner, New York, 1928
10. See also Hammonds, W.D. *Proc. 3rd Internat. Symp. Hist. Anaesth.* edited by B.R. Fink, L.E. Morris and C.R. Stephen, Wood Library-Museum of Anesthesiology, Park Ridge, Ill., 1992, pp.256–259; Papper, E.M. *ibid.*, pp.318–325
11. Gould, A.B. In *Anaesthesia; Essays in its History*, edited by J. Rupreht *et al.*, Springer-Verlag, Berlin, 1985, p.384
12. Vandam, L.D. and Abbott, J.A. *N. Engl. J. Med.*, 1984, **311**, 991
13. Bigelow, H.J. *Boston Med. Surg. J.*, 1846, **35**, 309 (reprinted in 'Classical File', *Surv. Anesthesiol.*, 1957, **1**, Feb.); Morton W.T.G. *Remarks on the*

Proper Mode of Administration of Sulphuric Ether by Inhalation, Dutton and Wentworth, 1847, Boston

14. Gould, A.B. In *Anaesthesia; Essays in its History,* edited by J. Rupreht *et al.*, Springer-Verlag, Berlin, 1985, p.384
15. Thomas, K. Bryn, *Anaesthesia,* 1968, **23**, 676
16. See also Keep, P. *Anaesthesia,* 1995, **50**, 233–238
17. Ellis, R.H. *Anaesthesia,* 1976, **31**, 766; *Anaesthesia,* 1977, **32**, 193; in *A History of Anaesthesia,* edited by R.S. Atkinson and T.B. Boulton, Royal Society of Medicine, London, 1989, p.69
18. Ellis, R.H. James Robinson: England's true pioneer of anaesthesia. In *Proc. 3rd Internat. Symp. Hist. Anaesth.,* edited by B.R. Fink, L.E. Morris and C.R. Stephen, Wood Library-Museum of Anesthesiology, Park Ridge, Ill., 1992
19. Editorial. Painless operations, *The Medical Times,* 1847, **15**, 328
20. Letter, Robinson, J. *The Medical Times,* 1847, **15**, 292
21. Boott, F. *Lancet,* 1847, **1**, 5–8
22. Annotation. *Anaesthesia,* 1984, **39**, 84
23. Dawkins, R.J. Massey. *Anaesthesia,* 1947, **2**, 51
24. Zuck, D. *Br. J. Anaesth.,* 1978, **50**, 393; Squire, W. *Lancet,* 1888, **2**, 1220
25. Baillie, T.W. *Br. J. Anaesth,* 1965, **37**, 952–957; *From Boston to Dumfries,* Dinwiddie, Dumfries, 1969
26. Secher, O., *Anaesthesia,* 1986, **41**, 829–837.
27. See Miller, A.H. *Boston Med. Surg. J.,* 1927, **197**, 1218; *Anesthesiology,* 1947, **8**, 471 (reprinted in 'Classical File', *Surv. Anesthesiol.,* 1972, **16**, 193); Straton, J. *Br. Med. J.,* 1972, **3**, 181
28. Miller, A.H. *Curr. Res. Anesth. Analg.* 1928, **7**, 240–247

3

Inhalation anaesthesia in the nineteenth century

Ether

Many different types of apparatus were designed to improve etherization within a few years of 1846. They tried to counter the problems of the cooling of the liquid ether that occurred as it evaporated, and the dilution of ether vapour that occurred with air. In 1847, several publications had appeared on the use of ether. Ether anaesthesia also immediately interested physiologists and other scientists, especially in France where Pierre Jean Marie Flourens (1794–1867), a Paris physiologist, concluded in 1847 that ether affected, in order as anaesthesia deepened, the higher cerebral centres, the cerebellum, the spinal cord and finally the medulla oblongata.[1] Flourens had previously demonstrated that the respiratory centres were located in the medulla.

John Snow (1813–58) (Figure 3.1), a London physician, was perhaps the most prominent doctor to apply scientific method to investigate the pharmacodynamics and clinical properties of ether. He became interested in ether soon after its introduction, and described five degrees of etherization in his publication of 1847:[2] *On the Inhalation of the Vapour of Ether in Surgical Operations*. The first three were of light anaesthesia, the fourth comprised what we would regard as surgical anaesthesia, and in the fifth respiration became progressively impaired.

Snow quickly perceived that the common method of administration was faulty, and devised several pieces of apparatus for delivering to the patient a known percentage concentration of anaesthetic vapour in an attempt to increase safety. He invented an ether inhaler in 1847 (Figure 3.2) and adapted the face-piece of Dr Francis Sibson (1816–76) of Nottingham. Later he invented his own face-piece. This work was stimulated by the first reports of deaths associated with anaesthesia. Two such deaths had been reported in March 1847, the first of a young woman at Grantham, Lincs, and the second a 52-year-old man at the Essex and Colchester Hospital.

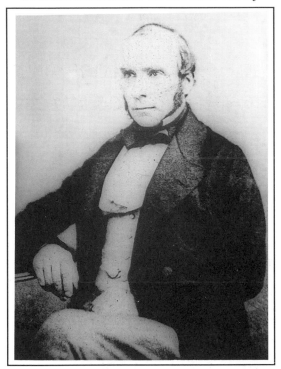

Figure 3.1　John Snow (1813–58)[3]

Born in York on 15 March 1813, the eldest of nine children of a farmer. After Morton, he was the first full-time anaesthetist. Starting his medical studies in Newcastle upon Tyne, at the age of 14, as apprentice to Mr William Hardcastle, he was one of the eight medical students who entered the Medical School, Newcastle upon Tyne, at its inception in 1832. Worked at the Newcastle Infirmary and became interested in the first cholera epidemic at Killingworth Colliery in 1831–32. In 1833 he left Newcastle and worked for a time as an assistant to Mr Watson at Burnop Field near Newcastle, and then under Mr Joseph Warburton at Pateley Bridge in Yorkshire. In 1836 he migrated to London, travelling on foot, and attended lectures at the Hunterian School of Anatomy in Great Windmill Street, founded by William Hunter (1718–84), elder brother of John Hunter (1728–92), and also at Westminster Hospital. Became a member of the Royal College of Surgeons of England in 1838 and also passed the examination of the Apothecaries Hall. Became MD, London, in 1844, and was appointed lecturer (1844–49) in forensic medicine at the Aldersgate School of Medicine just before its closure. After lodgings at Batemans Buildings, Soho, he set up practice at 54 Frith Street, where a commemorative plaque has now been erected,[4] and later at 18 Sackville Street in London, where he lived for the remainder of his life. He joined the Westminster Medical Society and wrote papers on many subjects, including resuscitation of the newborn[5] and paracentesis of the thorax.[6] Appointed anaesthetist to Out-Patients at St. George's Hospital, London, where his first anaesthetics (for dental extraction) were given, and later in 1847 was promoted to the

In-Patient appointment. Rapidly became the leading anaesthetist in London. Also worked with Robert Liston (1794–1847) at University College Hospital and with Sir William Fergusson (1808–77) at King's College Hospital. His health was poor and he suffered from phthisis and from nephritis, being treated for the latter by Richard Bright (1789–1858). For many years he was a vegetarian and an advocate of temperance. He experimented with many substances to see if they possessed anaesthetic properties, trying many of them on himself.

Snow came to prefer chloroform for use in adults, and gave over 4000 chloroform anaesthetics with only one possible death.[55] In 1853 he originated 'chloroform à la reine', when he acted as anaesthetist at the birth of the eighth child of Queen Victoria (1819–1901), Prince Leopold George Duncan Albert (1853–84), later the Duke of Albany who was to die of haemophilia. This administration of chloroform was at the request of Sir James Clark on 7 April 1853, and was repeated in 1857 at the birth of the Queen's last child, Princess Beatrice (1857–1944) on 14 April. These royal occasions made anaesthesia in midwifery morally and socially respectable, and canonized 'that blessed chloroform'. Gave his royal patient 15-minim doses intermittently on a handkerchief, the administration lasting 53 minutes. It met with the Queen's warm approval: 'Dr Snow gave that blissed chloroform . . . soothing quieting and delightful beyond measure.' Even the names of the Queen's attendants seemed to share the aura of purity which her royal participation had given to the subject: Mrs Lilly and Mrs Innocent the midwives, and of course Dr Snow![7] Snow's income never exceeded £1000 per annum, although during the last 10 years of his life he gave an average of 450 anaesthetics a year. His last work, *On Chloroform and Other Anaesthetics*, was published posthumously in 1858, as Snow was seized with paralysis while at work on the manuscript and died on 11 June 1858.

In his later years he achieved fame in a different field by proving that cholera is a water-borne disease, when he ordered the removal of the Broad Street (Golden Square) pump handle in 1854 in London. This action terminated the third cholera epidemic (although this particular epidemic had commenced to wane before the actual removal of the handle).[8] The theory of the mode of transmission of cholera was set out in the second edition of his book *On the Mode of Communication of Cholera*, 2nd edn, Churchill, London, 1855 (the first edition was published in 1849, following the epidemic of 1848 in which over 5000 people died). Snow's theories were substantiated by William Budd (1811–80).[9] It was, however, many years before Snow's views were generally accepted. Max von Pettenkoffer (1818–1901) was a leading anti-contagionist until his suicide in 1901. It is interesting that the cholera vibrio had been described in 1854 by Picini of Florence,[10] 30 years before Koch's paper.[11] Near the site of the pump, in Broadwick Street, a public house has been named 'The John Snow' (although Snow was a teetotaller!). His grave in Brompton Cemetery was restored in 1938 by anaesthetists from Britain and the USA. Benjamin Ward Richardson (1828–96)[12] wrote the epitaph which reads: 'In Brompton Cemetery there was laid to rest, at the age of forty-five, John Snow (1813–1858), exemplary citizen and useful physician. He demonstrated that cholera is communicated by contaminated water; and he made the art of anaesthesia a science.' The tombstone was destroyed by German bombing in April 1941, but was restored in 1950 and unveiled on 6 July 1951.[13] Three of his casebooks with a record of his chloroform administrations between 1848 and 1858 are in the possession of the Library of the Royal College of Physicians of London. The casebooks have been reproduced with a useful historical introduction.[14] The originals have been rebound, courtesy of the History of Anaesthesia Society.

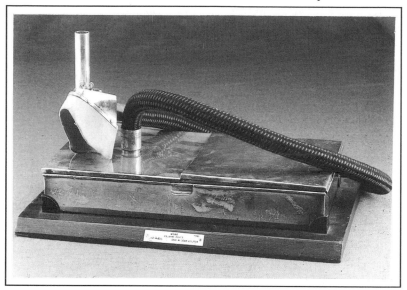

Figure 3.2   Snow's inhaler

Snow investigated many other potential volatile agents in the last 10 years of his life from 1848 to 1858. He was the first to realize the inverse relationship between solubility and potency. The agents he investigated included benzene, bromoform, ethyl bromide, ethyl nitrate, carbon disulphide, and lastly amylene (C_5H_{10}). Two patients died in 1857 while he was administering amylene to them. The first of these was just one week before he gave Queen Victoria chloroform for the second time at the birth of Princess Beatrice.

The work of Simpson (see below) and Snow was to ensure that chloroform became a favoured agent in Britain.   In his last publication John Snow wrote: 'I hold it, therefore, to be almost impossible that a death from this agent can occur in the hands of a medical man who is applying it with ordinary intelligence and attention.'[17] Ether did not regain much popularity in Britain until B. Joy Jeffries came from America and advocated ether as being safer than chloroform in 1872. Two years later Clover introduced his gas-ether sequence.[15] Ether became accepted as a safe all-purpose anaesthetic.[16]

The major advantages of ether over chloroform were: a relative lack of toxicity especially in light planes of anaesthesia; excellent muscle relaxation without severe respiratory depression; lack of cardiac depression even if overdosage had produced respiratory depression (which could readily be treated by positive pressure ventilation); relatively non-toxic products of metabolism (alcohol, acetaldehyde and acetic acid); and little tendency to cause dysrhythmias. The disadvantages of ether were: the risk of explosion and fire, although explosions have never been described during the administration of ether and air even when diathermy has been used; stimulation of the secretion of mucus; postoperative nausea and vomiting; and a slow induction and recovery due to its high solubility.

Chloroform

The anaesthetic properties of chloroform in animals were described by the previously mentioned Paris physiologist Pierre Flourens in 1847,[1] in a series of experiments in which he also used ethyl chloride as the sole anaesthetic agent. Chloroform had previously been identified in 1831 independently by Soubeiran (1793–1858), a Paris pharmacist, Justus von Liebig (1813–73), a Darmstadt chemist, and Samuel Guthrie (1782–1848), a chemist in Sackett's Harbour, New York State. Jean Baptiste Andre Dumas (1800–48), a Paris pharmacist, gave chloroform its name and wrote the first full description of its physical and chemical properties.

It had been used as a potential therapeutic agent for various diseases, and was suggested to James Young Simpson (1811–70) (Figure 3.3), the Professor of Midwifery at the University of Edinburgh, as a possible volatile anaesthetic agent by David Waldie (1813–89), the chemist at the Apothecaries' Company of Liverpool.[18] Waldie later felt that he never got the credit he deserved for the introduction of chloroform.

Chloroform was first used at St. Bartholomew's Hospital, London, under the name of 'chloric ether' by Sir William Lawrence (1783–1867) and Holmes Coote at the suggestion of Michael Cudmore Furnell in the spring of 1847,[19] some 6 months before Simpson first used it. However, its place in clinical practice was secured and popularized by Simpson who, with his two assistants James Mathews Duncan (1826–90) and George Keith, experimented by inhaling it themselves in Simpson's house, 52 Queen Street, Edinburgh on 4 November 1847. Four days later it was used clinically and a report was read to the Edinburgh Medical and Chirurgical Society on 10 November: 'Notice of a New Anaesthetic Agent as a Substitute for Sulphuric Ether in Surgery and Midwifery.' Chloroform was first given in London under its correct name, again at St. Bartholomew's Hospital, on 20 November 1847.[20]

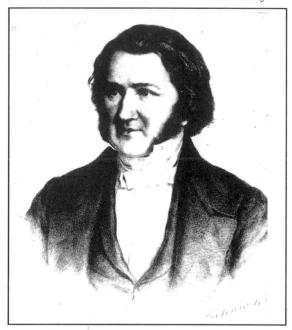

Figure 3.3 James Young Simpson (1811–70)[25]

Born at Bathgate, near Edinburgh. Qualified in 1830 and became M.D. in 1832. Elected to Chair of Midwifery at Edinburgh in 1840, spending £500 on canvassing, etc. Thus he started his university career in an atmosphere of hostility from his colleagues, but his ability as a lecturer soon attracted large classes of students. Simpson took an interest in a wide range of subjects, including leprosy, puerperal sepsis and hospital design. Put forward the method of haemostasis by acupressure to promote better wound healing. Made many contributions to the literature of archaeology, becoming President of the Society of Antiquaries of Scotland in 1861. He was made one of Her Majesty's Physicians in Scotland in 1847 and was created baronet in 1866. Was awarded an honorary doctorate at Oxford University, and was given the freedom of the city of Edinburgh. Also received many foreign honours. (When Simpson, on being awarded a baronetcy, was looking for a suitable crest, it was suggested that there should be a picture of a 'wee naked bairn' with the motto 'Does your mother know you're oot?')

Most famous for the introduction of chloroform in 1847.[20] It should be observed that Davy, Faraday, Hickman, Wells, Morton and Koller were all in their twenties when they made their discoveries. Simpson, however, was a veteran of 36! Was the first to introduce anaesthesia into obstetrics, and was harshly attacked more on moral than on theological grounds[26] (*Genesis*, chapter 3, verse 16) for using pain relief for women in labour.

From 1845 to his death in 1870, Simpson lived at 52 Queen Street, Edinburgh. The dining room has been preserved as 'The Discovery Room' and contains some of Simpson's furniture and possessions.[27] There is a memorial to Sir James Young Simpson in Westminster Abbey. He was buried in the family plot in Warriston Cemetery, Edinburgh.

Simpson had been impressed by ether, and had even been the first to use it in obstetric practice on 19 January 1847, but was seeking to overcome the technical difficulties associated with its administration. He had tried inhaling several organic vapours before using chloroform. He considered that chloroform had major advantages over ether: less was needed and it was therefore cheaper, it was more pleasant for the patient and induction was quicker. Chloroform was manufactured by Duncan Flockhart and Company (formerly Duncan, Anderson and Flockhart) of 52 North Bridge, Edinburgh. They became known worldwide and supplied chloroform during the Crimean War and the Franco-Prussian War of 1870.[21]

Snow, too, later abandoned ether for chloroform in adults, but was familiar with the dangers of the newer drug, believing it to cause primary cardiac failure if the vapour was too strong. To overcome this danger, Snow invented a percentage chloroform inhaler. For anaesthesia during labour, Snow poured a little chloroform on to a folded handkerchief, but for surgical operations he preferred the greater accuracy provided by his inhaler. In Scotland, the 'open method' originated by Simpson was the usual method of administration for both types of application. He poured drops of the newer agent on to gauze held near the face of the patient, so avoiding the use of the inhalers which were used for ether. Thomas Skinner, a Liverpool obstetrician, developed a gauze-covered mask for this purpose which was adapted by Curt Schimmelbusch (1860–95), a German surgeon.

Within a few months chloroform superseded ether as the most popular anaesthetic agent in Britain. The first reported death due to chloroform was that of 15-year-old Hannah Greener of Winlayton, near Newcastle upon Tyne, little more than two months after its introduction (28 January 1848). The anaesthetic was given for a minor operation by Dr Meggison. John Snow gave over 4000 chloroform anaesthetics with only one possible death and, early on, recommended that for safety a concentration of not more than 4% in air should be used. Following 1890, reports of liver damage appeared in the literature.[22]

The problem of toxicity with chloroform was to lead to its loss of favour in England and much later in Scotland (it was still being given in Scotland in the 1970s). The blood pressure gradually fell with deepening anaesthesia. Sudden cardiac arrest, occurring during light anaesthesia,[23] was due to ventricular fibrillation or vagal inhibition. Ventricular fibrillation during light chloroform anaesthesia had been shown by Goodman Levy (1856–1954) in 1911.[24] Rarely, chloroform damaged the liver, and the presentation of this was delayed to between the first and third day after anaesthesia. It was more likely to follow repeated administrations.

The first major war in which anaesthetics were used was the Crimean War (1854–55). It is an interesting fact, however, that even as long as 25 years after Morton introduced the use of ether in surgery, operations were still being performed in the complete absence of any form of anaesthesia, even in European teaching hospitals.[28] Different uses of ether and chloroform, and different methods of administration, were adopted in different countries. Thus chloroform was used more frequently in Scotland, the greater part of Europe and in the southern states of America, while ether remained the favourite in England and in the northern states of America. There was much controversy as to which was the safer of the two drugs. Concern over deaths apparently associated with the use of chloroform prompted the Royal Medical and Chirurgical Society to appoint a committee to investigate. Its report in 1864[29] drew attention to the dangers of chloroform, but considered ether to be impractical because of the lengthy induction and prolonged excitatory phase. It recommended the use of mixtures of ether and chloroform, and many anaesthetists either used these or increasingly used chloroform for induction and then switched to ether for maintenance. In around 1860 George Harley had introduced the ACE mixture (alcohol, chloroform and ether in the ratio 1:2:3), which gained considerable acceptance. These were important new concepts. They suggested that it was unprofitable to search for the perfect universal agent, and that different anaesthetics may be needed at different stages of an operation.

By the 1870s ether had largely won the day, except perhaps in obstetric analgesia. When John Snow, England's leading physician anaesthetist, died in 1858, his place was taken by Joseph Thomas Clover (1825–82)* who took on the mantle of the country's leading

---

* Joseph Thomas Clover (1825–82)[30] (see fig 16.1)

Born in Aylesham, Norfolk and educated at the Greyfriars' Priory School in Norwich and at University College Hospital in London (1844). It is possible, although some feel it unlikely,[31] that he was actually present at the operating theatre at University College Hospital for the first ether anaesthetic in England (21 December 1846). Nevertheless he was interested in anaesthesia from its beginning. Joseph Lister (1827–1912) was a fellow student. Became house surgeon to James Syme (1799–1870) and later RMO at University College Hospital and took FRCS in 1850. Pioneer of the art of completely and immediately removing from the urinary bladder the calculus fragments produced by lithotrity and invented a bladder aspirator, the forerunner of Bigelow's evacuator (1878). Also devised 'Clover's crutch', a simple but effective piece of apparatus for maintaining a patient in the lithotomy position. Because of poor health, he worked as general practitioner in London in 1853, later specializing in anaesthetics, thereby helping to fill the vacancy created by the early death of John

Snow in 1858. Appointed to the staff of University College and Westminster Hospitals, and also worked at the London Dental Hospital. For many years he was the leading anaesthetist in London. Between 1853 and his death in 1882 he lived at 3 Cavendish Place, the site now commemorated by a plaque. Attended many famous people, including the ex-Emperor Napoleon III of France (1808–73) at Chislehurst where he was operated on three times in 1871, the Princess of Wales (later Queen Alexandra), Sir Robert Peel and Miss Florence Nightingale. Never a man of robust constitution, he died at the age of 57.[32] Eleven years before his death he was to claim that he had had no deaths in 11 000 administrations, 7000 of them using chloroform.[33] Unfortunately, he had one death later.[34] An eponymous lecture is given every two years in his honour, alternately with a similar lecture honouring the name of Frederick Hewitt, at the Royal College of Anaesthetists in London. His figure is depicted on the left side of the College coat of arms. Buried in Brompton Cemetery, London, his grave (No. U 113122) being 200 yards from that of John Snow.

---

scientific anaesthetic investigator and practical anaesthetist. Partly due to the influence of these two pioneers, the administration of anaesthetics in Britain has always been in the hands of medical men and, as time has passed, in the hands of specialists in the subject.

In 1862 Clover invented a chloroform inhaler which enabled percentage mixtures of chloroform and air to be accurately measured and administered. This took the form of a large bag, slung over the back of the anaesthetist, and containing 4.5% of chloroform vapour in air. Clover was co-opted on to the committee which investigated chloroform, realized its dangers, and set to work to make the administration of ether simpler and easier. He later worked on inducing anaesthesia with nitrous oxide, before later adding ether to the gas, and described the first apparatus for such sequential administration.[35] In 1877 he described his portable regulating ether inhaler[36] which did much to make ether more popular at the expense of chloroform. The inhaler of French surgeon Louis Ombrédanne (1871–1956)[37] was a slightly modified copy, using a pig's bladder instead of a rubber bag.[38] Another of Clover's achievements was his teaching that ether could be safely given over long periods with anaesthesia carried to adequate depth.

Nitrous oxide

Despite the pre-eminence of ether, nitrous oxide still had its friends in the USA, and from 1863 to 1868 Gardner Colton, who had originally introduced it to Wells, embarked on a campaign to popularize the gas. This time the American dental profession showed considerable interest. In 1863 Colton established himself in practice in New York City and there founded the Colton Dental Association. T. W. Evans (1823–97), an American dentist working in Paris, introduced it to his colleagues in London in 1868,[39] having learnt its use the previous year from Colton at the International Congress of Medicine in Paris.

Its main disadvantages were the difficulty in administration and the asphyxia which was inseparable from its use as pure nitrous oxide. In late 1868 the gas was supplied compressed into cylinders (Barth, and then Coxeter & Son, in London) and became available two years later as liquefied nitrous oxide. A reducing valve was described in 1873. The asphyxia was partly overcome by Edmund Andrews (1824–1904) of Chicago who in 1868 gave it with 20% oxygen so as to allow prolonged anaesthesia.[40] Also in 1868, Clover proved nitrous oxide to be a true anaesthetic, not working merely by causing asphyxia. He successfully demonstrated its use at a meeting of the British Medical Association at the Radcliffe Infirmary, Oxford.[41] He published an influential paper 'On the Administration of Nitrous Oxide' later that year.[42]

Clover also introduced the nitrous oxide–ether sequence in 1876,[43] and early users of the nitrous oxide (with oxygen)–chloroform/ether sequence were F. J. Cotton (1869–1938); W. M. Boothby (1880–1953) of Boston; J. T. Gwathmey (1863–1944) of New York City; Geoffrey Marshall (1887–1982) and H. E. G. Boyle (1875–1941) of London.[44] In 1878 Paul Bert (1830–86), of France, administered nitrous oxide in a hyperbaric chamber, and designed a mobile pressurized operating theatre which he took around the hospitals of Paris.[45] Bert was also an early user of Andrews's nitrous oxide–oxygen mixture.[46]

Amylene

Of particular interest because it was used successfully by Snow on many occasions,[47] amylene was later abandoned following two deaths, one of which occurred only one week before his second administration of chloroform to Queen Victoria.[48]

Ethyl chloride

This was the last general anaesthetic agent of any importance to be introduced in the nineteenth century. Its efficacy had been shown in animals by P. J. M. Flourens in 1847 during the course of his experiments on chloroform[1], and confirmed clinically in 1848 by J. F. Heyfelder at Erlangen in Germany. He noted its rapid action and relative freedom from side-effects, but the pure chemical was difficult to obtain, and of course it was highly volatile. During 1890 and 1891, it became available from a French company, and Redard of Geneva introduced ethyl chloride as a local anaesthetic spray, especially for dentistry. It was used in England at King's College Hospital by Underwood.[49] By 1894 this use by dental surgeons had resulted in accidental general anaesthesia, and the apparent ease of use led some to adopt it for this purpose. The first death associated with its use was in 1899 at Professor von Hacker's department of surgery at the Sophien Hospital, Vienna.

Its use in England was encouraged in 1901 by William J. McCardie, an anaesthetist at Birmingham,[50] and in America by Martin W. Ware, surgeon in New York.[51] Several anaesthetists used ethyl chloride just for induction, and then changed to ether or chloroform for maintenance, as its dangers soon became apparent.

The close of the nineteenth century

After this rush of innovation the development of anaesthesia became less dramatic, with significant advances interrupting periods of stagnation. Parallel with the development of anaesthesia, but delayed by a few years, was the introduction of antiseptic methods of surgery. The combination of antisepsis and anaesthesia allowed the development of prolonged and delicate surgery that could not have been conceived in the first half of the century. This was eventually to convince even the most diehard surgeon that anaesthesia was a discipline that demanded its own specialist, who could choose the agents and apparatus most suited to the patient, his or her condition and the proposed surgery, and who was skilled in their administration. This realization came first in Britain and in America, and rather later on the continent of Europe.

For the further development of anaesthesia in the USA, see Waters, R. M. (1946) *J. Hist. Med. Allied Sci.*, **1**, 595; and Eckenhoff, J. E. (1978) *Anesthesiology*, **49**, 272.

For the introduction of anaesthesia into:

France (by Jobert de Lamballe and J. F. Malgaigne at the Hôpital St. Louis, Paris), see Neveu, R. *J. Hist. Med. Allied Sci.*, 1946, **1**, 607.

Germany (by Heyfelder of Erlangen), see Frankel, W. K. *J. Hist. Med. Allied Sci.*, 1946, **1**, 612; Whitacre, R. J. and Dumitra, J. H. M. *J. Hist. Med. Allied Sci.*, 1946, **1**, 618; von Hintzenstern, U. In *A History of Anaesthesia*, edited by R. S. Atkinson and T. B. Boulton, Royal Society of Medicine, London, 1989, p.502. For the further early development of anaesthesiology as a speciality in Germany, see Schwarz, W. In *A History of Anaesthesia*, edited by R.S. Atkinson and T. B. Boulton, Royal Society of Medicine, London, 1989, p.170.

The Netherlands, see van Wijhe, M, *From Stupefaction to Narcosis,* Slinger, Alkmaar, 1991. Also see Vermeulen-Cranch, D. In *Anaesthesia: Essays on its History,* edited by J. Rupreht *et al.*; Springer-Verlag, Berlin, 1985, p.156. Also, Rupreht, J. In *A History of Anaesthesia,* edited by R.S. Atkinson and T. B. Boulton, Royal Society of Medicine, London, 1989, p.86.

New Zealand, where the first anaesthetic (for a dental extraction) was given by Mr Marriott with Dr J. P. Fitzgerald as surgeon, see Newson, A. J. *Anaesth. Intensive Care,* 1975, **3**, 204.

Australia, where the first anaesthetic was given by Dr Wm Russ Pugh of Tasmania on 7 June 1847.[52] The first anaesthetic in Melbourne, Victoria was given on 2 July 1847 and in Adelaide, South Australia by Kent on 30 September 1847.[53]

The Australian Society of Anaesthetists was founded in 1934. An account of the history of the Australian Society of Anaesthetists by G. C. Wilson was published in 1987.[54] The Faculty of Anaesthetists of the Royal Australian College of Surgeons was founded in 1952, with the first fellowship examination in 1956. It is now the Australian and New Zealand College of Anaesthetists.

Republic of South Africa, see Kok, O. V. S. *Progress in Anaesthesiol.* Proc. 4th World Congress Anaes., Amsterdam, Excerpta Medica, 1970, p.167; and also Cooper, J. L. In *A History of Anaesthesia,* edited by R. S. Atkinson and T. B. Boulton, Royal Society of Medicine, London, 1989, p.147.

Canada, see Matsuki, A. *Can. Anaesth. Soc. J.,* 1974, **21**, 92; and also Maltby, J. R. In *A History of Anaesthesia,* edited by R. S. Atkinson and T. B. Boulton, Royal Society of Medicine, London, 1989, p.112.

Argentina, see Cooper, I. *Br. Med. Bull.,* 1946, **4**, 147.

For the development of anaesthesia in other countries see *Anaesthesia: Essays on its History,* edited by J. Rupreht *et al.* Springer-Verlag, Berlin, 1985. Countries, with page numbers: **Czechoslovakia** (Dworacek, B. and Keszler, H.), 41; **Italy** (Pantaleoni, M.), 113; **Ecuador** (Pinto, O. M.), 115; **Japan** (Yamamura, H.), 165; **China** (Shieh Yung), 136; **Yugoslavia** (Darinka Sobin), 139; **Nigeria** (Sodipo, J. O. A.), 141; **Ukraine** (Treshchinsky, A. I.), 153; **Thailand** (Tupavong, S.), 154; **Lebanon** (Haddad, F. S.), 60; **Spain** (Franco, A., Ginesta, M. V. *et al.*), 48; **Hungary** (Forgacs, I. and Varga, P.), 45; **Russia** (Damir, E.), 28. Also, in *A History of Anaesthesia,* edited by R. S. Atkinson and T. B. Boulton, Royal Society of Medicine, London, 1989, with page numbers: **Hong Kong** (Lett, Z.), 153; **California** (Calmes, S. H.) 129.

For documentation of 46 'first anaesthetics' in the world, see Secher, O., *Acta Anaesthesiol. Scand.*, 1990, **34**, 55.

References

1. Flourens, P.J.M. *C.R. Acad. Sci. Paris*, 1847, **24**, 161, 253, 340
2. Reprinted in *Br. J. Anaesth.*, 1953, **25**, 53–67, 162–169, 253–267, 349–382
3. See also John Snow; first anaesthetist, *Bios*, 1936, **7**, 25; Keys, T.E. John Snow: Anaesthetist, *J. Hist. Med. Allied Sci.*, 1946, **1**, 551–556; Sir Benjamin Ward Richardson, John Snow: biography, reprinted in *Br. J. Anaesth.*, 1952, **24**, 267; Snow on the water of London, *Mayo Clin. Proc.*, 1974, **49**, 480; Lord Cohen of Birkenhead, John Snow – the autumn loiterer, *Proc. R. Soc. Med.* 1969, **62**, 99; Leaman, A. John Snow MD. His early days, *Anaesthesia*, 1984, **39**, 803–805; John Snow, *On Narcotism by the Inhalation of Vapours*, Royal Society of Medicine, London, 1991; Shephard, D.A.E. *John Snow. Anaesthetist to a Queen and Epidemiologist to a Nation. A Biography*, York Point Publishing, Cornwall, Prince Edward Island, Canada, 1995.
4. Ellis, R.H. In *A History of Anaesthesia*, edited by R. S. Atkinson and T. B. Boulton, Royal Society of Medicine, London, 1989
5. Snow, J. *London Med. Gaz.*, 1841, **29**, 222–227
6. Snow, J. *London Med. Gaz.*, 1842, **29**, 705–707
7. Longford, E. *Victoria R. I.*, Weidenfeld and Nicolson, London, 1964, p.234
8. Winterton, W.R. *Hist. Med.*, 1980, **8**, 11; Schoenberg, B.S. *et al. Mayo Clinic Proc.*, 1974, **49**, 680
9. Budd, W. Malignant cholera: its mode of propagation, and its prevention, *Lond. Med. Gaz.* 1849, **44**, 724
10. Picini, F. *Osservazioni microscopische e deduction patologische sul cholera asiatica*, Firenze, 1854
11. Koch, R. Ueber die cholera bakterien. *Dtsch. Med. Wochenschr*, 1884, **10**, 725
12. *Br. J. Anaesth.*, 1955, **27**, 517
13. *Anaesthesia* ,1952, **7**, 192
14. Ellis, R. H. (ed.) *The Casebooks of Dr John Snow*, Wellcome Institute for the History of Medicine, 1995
15. Clover, J.T. *Med. Times Lond.*, 1874, **2**, 603; Vandam, L. *Anesthesiology*, 1980, **52**, 62
16. Epstein, H. G. and Macintosh, R. R. *Anaesthesia*, 1956, **11**, 83; Farman, J. V. *Anaesthesia and the EMO System*, English Universities Press, London, 1973
17. John Snow, *On Chloroform and Other Anaesthetics*, 1858
18. Waldie, D., *The True Story of the Introduction of Chloroform into Anaesthetics*, Linlithgow, Edinburgh, 1870
19. Furnell, M.C. *Lancet*, 1871, **1**, 433; *ibid.* 1877, **1**, 934
20. Simpson, J.Y. *Lond. Med. Gaz.*, 1847, **5**, 934; *Lancet*, 1847, **2**, 549; reprinted in *Foundations of Anesthesiology*, Vol. 1, edited by A. Faulcolner and T. E. Keys, Thomas, Springfield, Ill, p.463; also in 'Classical File', *Surv. Anesthesiol.*, 1961, **5**, 93; Sykes, W. S. *Essays on the First*

Hundred Years of Anaesthesia, Vol. II, Livingstone, Edinburgh, 1961, p.168; Coote, H. *Lancet,* 1847, **2,** 571

21. Atkinson, R. S. *James Simpson and Chloroform,* Priory Press, London, 1973

22. Guthrie, L. *Lancet,* 1894, **1,** 193, 257; 1903, **2,** 10 (reprinted in 'Classical File', *Surv. Anesthesiol.,* 1962, **6,** 422)

23. *Proc. R. Soc. Med.,* 1914, **7,** 57 (reprinted in 'Classical File', *Surv. Anesthesiol.,* 1973, **17,** 383)

24. Levy, A. G. *Chloroform Anaesthesia.,* Bale Son and Daniellson, London, 1922; *Proc. R. Soc. Med.,* 1914, **7,** 57 (reprinted in 'Classical File', *Surv. Anesthesiol.,* 1973, **17,** 383 and 477)

25. See also Shepherd, J. A. *Simpson and Syme of Edinburgh.* Livingstone, 1969; Edinburgh; Simpson, Myrtle. *Simpson the Obstetrician.,* Gollancz, London, 1972

26. Farr, A. D. *Anaesthesia,* 1980, **35,** 896

27. Atkinson, R. S. (1973) *Simpson and Chloroform,* Priory Press, London, 1973; *Anaesthesia,* 1973, **28,** 302

28. *Med. Times Lond.,* 1868, **2,** 9; Pernick, M. S. *A Calculus of Suffering,* Columbia University Press, New York, 1985

29. *Medico-chirurgical Transactions,* 1864, **47,** 323–442

30. See Calverley, R. In *Anaesthesia, Essays on its History,* edited by J. Rupreht *et al.,* Springer-Verlag, Berlin, 1985, p.18; Woollam, C. H. M. *Curr. Anaesth. Crit. Care,* 1994, **5,** 53–61; Adams, A. K. *Proc. Hist. Anaesth. Soc.,* 1989, **6A,** 50–52 and **7,** 7–10

31. Thomas K. Bryn. *Anaesthesia,* 1971, **27,** 436

32. Lee, J. A. *Ann. R. Coll. Surg.,* 1960, **26,** 280; Wylie, W. D. *Ann. R. Coll. Surg.,* 1975, **56,** 171

33. Clover, J. T. *Br. Med. J.,* 1871, **2,** 33

34. Clover, J. T. *Br. Med. J.,* 1874, **1,** 817–818

35. Clover, J. T. *Br. Med. J.,* 1876, **2,** 74 (reprinted in 'Classical File', *Surv. Anesthesiol.,* 1964, **8,** 87)

36. Clover, J. T. *Br. Med. J.,* 1877, **1,** 69–70; Atkinson, R. S. and Boulton, T. B. *Anaesthesia,* 1977, **32,** 1033

37. L'Anaesthésie par l'Ether, *Gazette des Hospit.,* 1908, 1095

38. Elliott, C. J. R. *Anaesthesia,* 1979, **34,** 681; Brown, A. G. *Anaesthesia,* 1979, **34,** 681; Weisser, Ch. *Anaesthesist,* 1983, **32,** 52

39. Evans, T. W. *Br. J. Dent. Sci.,* 1868, **2,** 196

40. Andrews, E. A. *Chicago Med. Examiner,* 1868, **19,** 656 (reprinted in 'Classical File', *Surv. Anesthesiol.,* 1963, **7,** 74)

41. Clover, J. T. *Br. Med. J.,* 1868, **2,** 201

42. Clover, J. T. *Br. Med. J.,* 1868, **2,** 491

43. Clover, J. T. *Br. Med. J.,* 1876, **2,** 74 (reprinted in 'Classical File', *Surv. Anesthesiol.,* 1964, **8,** 87)

44. Boulton, T. B. 'Classical File', *Surv. Anesthesiol.,* 1985, **29,** 201; *ibid.,* 1992, **36,** 40–49

45. Bert, P. *C.R.. Soc. Biol. Paris,* 1878, **87,** 728; *ibid.,* 1879, **89,** 132

46. Bert, P. *C.R. Acad. Sci. Paris,* 1883, **96,** 1271

47. Snow, J. On the vapour of amylene, *Med. Times Gaz.*, 1857, ns 14, 60–62 and 82–84; Further remarks on amylene, *ibid.* pp.332–334 and 357–359

48. Snow, J. Further remarks on amylene: instance of death from that agent, *Med. Times Gaz.*, 1857, ns 14, 379–382; Case of death from amylene, *ibid.*, 1857, ns 15, 133–134; see also Conacher, I.D. *Anaesthesia*, 1996, **51**, 155

49. *J. Br. Dent. Assoc.*, 1891, **12**, 780

50. Annotation, *Lancet*, 1901, **i**, 698

51. Annotation, *Med. News N. Y.*, 1904, **84**, 1026

52. Wilson, G. C. *Anaesth. Intensive Care*, 1985, **13**, 71

53. Wilson, G. C. *Anaesth. Intensive Care*, 1987, **15**, 451; Schurr, P. H. *Benjamin's Son*, Royal Society of Medicine, London, 1991

54. Wilson, G. C. *Fifty Years*, The Australian Society of Anaesthetists, Flannel Flower Press, Glebe, NSW, 1987 and Wilson, GC. *One grand chain*, Vol. 1 pp 1846–1934, Australian and New Zealand College of Anaesthetists, Melbourne, Vic, 1995.

55. Snow, J. *Med. Times. Gaz.*, 1852, **5**, 361–362.

4
Developments in the twentieth century

During the late 1800s and early 1900s there were few significant changes in inhalation anaesthesia – it was more a period of consolidation. At the turn of the century two German pharmacologists, Hans Meyer (1853–1939) of Vienna and Charles Overton (1865–1933) of Zurich, proposed that inhalational anaesthetic potency increased with lipid solubility.[1] This hypothesis has proved to be fairly robust, presumably since anaesthetic agents act on the brain, which is rich in lipid.

Two important textbooks appeared for the first time in the late nineteenth century, which helped uphold the standard of British anaesthesia which faced a significant void after Clover died in 1882. In 1888 Dudley Wilmot Buxton, anaesthetist at University College Hospital, London, published *Anaesthetics: their Uses and Administration*, and in 1893 Frederick W. Hewitt (1857–1916) (Figure 4.1) published *Anaesthetics and their Administration*. Both these books ran to many editions, and their influence was widespread. Buxton's book included a chapter on the medico-legal aspects of the administration of anaesthetics. The fifth edition of Hewitt's book was published in 1922. Hewitt emphasized that nitrous oxide anaesthesia is possible without asphyxia and that chloroform is especially dangerous during induction.

Hewitt[2] and later E. I. McKesson (1881–1935) (also an early pioneer of careful notekeeping in anaesthesia)[3] were pioneers in the use of nitrous oxide. Two books were published in 1939 on nitrous oxide: *Nitrous Oxide–Oxygen Anesthesia* by F. W. Clement (1892–1970), and *Untoward Effects of Nitrous Oxide Anaesthesia* by C. B. Courville, a Los Angeles neuropathologist. The latter dealt with acute asphyxia caused by McKesson's technique of secondary saturation.

At this time, ether and chloroform were still the main agents, but ethyl chloride and nitrous oxide were often used for induction. Simpson's open drop method was the most popular, while the first Boyle machine appeared in 1917. From this time onwards the pace

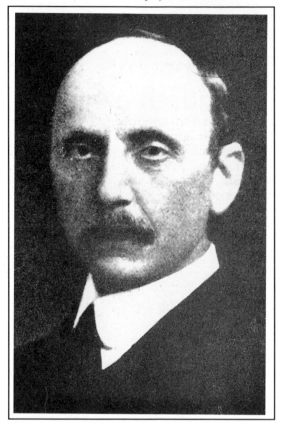

Figure 4.1 Sir Frederick W. Hewitt (1857–1916)

Educated at Merchant Taylors' School, Christ's College, Cambridge, and St. George's Hospital, London, where he was a distinguished student. Defective eyesight prevented his becoming a consulting physician, and so he turned to anaesthesia and was appointed to Charing Cross Hospital in this capacity in 1884, the National Dental Hospital in 1885, and lecturer on anaesthesia at the London Hospital in 1886. In 1902 he became physician anaesthetist to his old teaching hospital, St. George's. Hewitt modified Junker's chloroform bottle and redesigned Clover's inhaler, enlarging the bore of the central tube, as suggested by Wilson Smith,[4] and arranging for its rotation within the ether reservoir. He also devised an airway[5] and a dental prop. Strongly advocated better teaching of anaesthetics to medical students. A superb clinical anaesthetist, he was a tireless advocate for greater care to be taken in the administration of anaesthetics and constantly sought to improve conditions under which anaesthetics were given, and to protect the public against their use by unqualified persons. Persuaded the government to draft a Bill to outlaw the administration of anaesthetics by unqualified people, although World War I prevented its passage.[6] Invented the first practical machine for giving nitrous oxide and oxygen in fixed proportions in 1887. Administered anaesthesia to Edward VII for drainage of an appendix abscess on 27 June 1902,[7] two days before his coronation was due. The ceremony then took place on 9 August 1902. Sir Frederick Treves (1853–1916) was the surgeon. Hewitt was knighted in 1911 and died in Brighton in 1916 of a gastric neoplasm. His grave lies in Brighton and Preston Cemetery.[8] An eponymous lecture in his honour is given every two years by the Royal College of Anaesthetists in London.

---

of progress quickened, and has continued to do so ever since. Before the 1930s the anaesthetist administered one or two volatile agents which produced unconsciousness, muscle relaxation and deafferentation. This method gave place to various techniques of so-called 'balanced anaesthesia' and so the amount of toxic drugs to which the patient was exposed was reduced and the hazards of anaesthesia lessened.

The concept of balanced anaesthesia started in 1911 when George Washington Crile (1864–1943) of Cleveland, Ohio, taught that 'psychic stimuli' must be obliterated by light general anaesthesia, while the noxious impulses due to surgery must be blocked by local analgesia, the so-called theory of anoci-association.[9] In 1926 John S. Lundy (1894–1972) of the Mayo Clinic introduced the term 'balanced anaesthesia' for a combination of agents such as premedication, regional analgesia and general anaesthesia with one or more agents, so that pain relief was obtained by a judicious mix of agents and techniques.[10] Rees and Gray[11] from Liverpool divided anaesthesia into three basic components: narcosis, analgesia and relaxation. Gray renamed[12] this the 'triad' of narcosis, reflex suppression and relaxation.

Among other innovations were the popularization of endotracheal techniques by Ivan W. Magill and E. Stanley Rowbotham (1890–1979),[13] the appearance of bromethol (Avertin), divinyl ether, cyclopropane and trichloroethylene, and the induction of anaesthesia by intravenous barbiturates in the early 1930s. Because of the difficulty of obtaining relaxation of the jaw and larynx with ether, blind nasotracheal intubation became increasingly used. Controlled respiration was used with cyclopropane so that when curare was first tried out by Harold Griffith in Montreal in 1942, the way to deal with hypoventilation and apnoea was well established, and soon intermittent positive pressure ventilation became routine practice.

Both the two world wars were to force the rate of change for surgery and anaesthesia. Following each war a number of doctors continued their anaesthetic work, which had been learnt under service conditions, into civilian life. They had a considerable influence on the development of the speciality.

Technical improvements in anaesthesia and the administration of anaesthetics were slowly accompanied by academic recognition, but

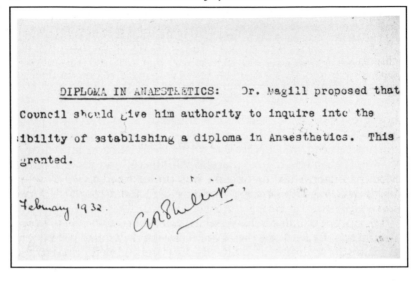

DIPLOMA IN ANAESTHETICS: Dr. Magill proposed that Council should give him authority to inquire into the ibility of establishing a diploma in Anaesthetics. This granted.

February 19 32

Figure 4.2 Section of anaesthetics of the Royal Society of Medicine minute about the Diploma in Anaesthesia

not always by adequate financial rewards. The first examination for the Diploma in Anaesthesia was held in London in 1935 (Figure 4.2). This was historically very significant because it enabled anaesthesia to become a speciality in its own right, the opening of a door through which improvement of standards and techniques were to flow in the succeeding decades. (The College of Surgeons had made a similar step in the early nineteenth century). Francis McMechan was engineering a parallel development in the USA in the 1930s. Other specialities are now in a similar position to anaesthesia in the 1930s. So the evolution of medicine continues!

The first university chair of anaesthesia was created at the University of Wisconsin in Madison in the USA in 1933. Ralph Waters was appointed as the first professor of anaesthesia there. The first chair of anaesthesia in Britain was created in Oxford in 1937,[14] with R. R. Macintosh as professor. In the UK the recognition of anaesthesia as a speciality with full equality with other medical and surgical specialities was secured in 1948 with the introduction of the National Health Service, and since then anaesthesia has not only kept pace with the rapid advances made in surgery, but has in many instances enabled these advances to be made. In recent decades the scope of the anaesthetist's work has widened, and now takes in not only preoperative assessment and postoperative care, but supervision of intensive therapy units, pain clinics, and in many cases research and postgraduate education. An enormous development in the use of highly sophisticated monitoring equipment has taken place in the past 20 years. Among those workers who remember clinical anaesthesia in the 1930s and early 1940s, few would disagree with the statement that what is known as 'modern anaesthesia' commenced with the introduction of the muscle relaxants.

General comments

Modern medical use of oxygen was popularized in 1917 by J. S. Haldane (1860–1936) during World War I,[15] and by Yandell Henderson, the New Haven physiologist (1873–1944).

Medical (and industrial) oxygen was later to be manufactured by the fractional distillation of liquid air, patented by Carl Linde of Germany. The boiling point of oxygen is −183°C. The oxygen concentrator is suitable for home use or where cylinders are unavailable.[16]

Helium was isolated in 1895 by Sir W. Ramsey (1852–1916), the British chemist and Nobel prizewinner in 1904 for his work on the inert gases.

The stimulating effect of carbon dioxide on respiration was shown by Herman and Escher in 1870,[17] and it became used by anaesthetists for this purpose soon after the work of Haggard and Yandell Henderson[18] in the USA (1921) who recommended 5% CO_2 in oxygen. However, fatal accidents have occurred with accidental overdosage.[19]

Another early pioneer in the USA was Arthur Guedel (1883–1956) (Figure 4.3) who made many important contributions to the development of the speciality.

The ill-effects of inadequate ventilation were thought to be due to hypoxia until Ralph Milton Waters (1883–1979) (Figure 4.4), then in private practice in Sioux City, Iowa, pointed out the possibility of CO_2 excess in the late 1920s.[20] He realized that the respired CO_2 could be controlled, at least in anaesthetized animals, following the work of D. E. Jackson, a Cincinnati pharmacologist.[21] Waters also deliberately used 30% carbon dioxide to render humans unconscious in 1928, echoing Henry Hill Hickman's work.[22]

Carbon dioxide absorption during anaesthesia was pioneered by John Snow, but extensively developed by Waters, whose first reason for the use of CO_2 absorption was economy and convenience (even more important when he started to use cyclopropane). After relaxants were introduced and IPPV became commonplace, hypocapnia was readily produced. This was originally thought to be harmless or

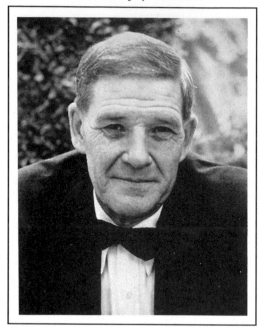

Figure 4.3   Arthur E. Guedel (1883–1956)[32]

Born in Cambridge City, Indiana, and received his medical education at the Indiana School of Medicine, Indianapolis, qualifying in 1908. Lost three fingers of his right hand at aged 13, but nevertheless became a skilled pianist. Started as a general practitioner and anaesthetist. Became lecturer on anaesthesia in the University of Indianapolis (1920–28), during which time he was a practising anaesthetist in that city. Gave anaesthetics in France during World War I (1917–19) and made notes on which he based a book. Later moved to Los Angeles, where he became associate clinical professor of anesthesiology at the University of Southern California School of Medicine. A leading pioneer of American anaesthesia, and like most of his contemporaries in the speciality he was self-taught.

Made many contributions to his chosen speciality, including an early description of the self-administration of nitrous oxide and air for obstetrics and minor surgery;[33] a description of the anaesthetic properties of divinyl ether; reintroduction, with R. M. Waters, of a cuffed tracheal tube;[34] a systemization of the signs of inhalation anaesthesia;[35] a pharyngeal airway;[36] the introduction of controlled respiration using ether, with Treweek;[37] and a classic description of the clinical use of cyclopropane.[38] Received the Hickman Medal from the Royal Society of Medicine in 1941, and the Distinguished Service Award of the American Society of Anesthesiologists in 1951. There is a Guedel Memorial Anesthesia Center in San Francisco, together with an eponymous lecture established in his honour by the University of California Medical Center in Los Angeles.

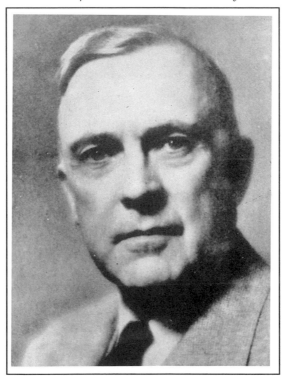

Figure 4.4   Ralph Milton Waters (1883–1979)

Born in North Bloomfield, Ohio, of Anglo-Scottish descent. Became a student at Western Reserve University in Cleveland in 1903 and after taking an arts degree became MD in 1912. Settled in general practice in Sioux City, Iowa, married and remained there for 5 years. Gradually became interested in anaesthesia and the basic sciences so that by 1916 anaesthesia came to occupy much of his time and he decided to specialize: an unusual step to take at the time. Opened a private clinic as a commercial venture with an operating room and facilities for minor surgery, where he gave the anaesthetics – one of the first day-stay clinics in the USA. In 1923, acquired an anaesthetic practice in Kansas City where he remained for 3 years. Hurt his back lifting an overweight patient, and as a result had to spend 6 months in a brace. On recovery he visited John S. Lundy (1884–1973), chief anaesthetist at the Mayo Clinic, and on his way home stopped off with friends at Madison. Here he met Chauncey Leake (1896–1978) the pharmacologist, and Erwin Schmidt, professor of surgery, and as a result was invited in 1927 to take charge of anaesthesia at the new Hospital of the State of Wisconsin at Madison which opened in 1924. Became in turn assistant professor, associate professor and, in 1933, full professor of anaesthesia with clinical charge of anaesthesia in the university hospitals. This was the first such post in the USA. Established the first resident training programme in anaesthesia.

Had a long and distinguished career and his clinic became one of the leading centres of anaesthesia in the world. Visited Europe and the UK in 1936. Was awarded the Hickman Medal by the Royal Society of Medicine in London in 1938, the first worker outside the UK to be so honoured. Retired in 1949 and was succeeded by Alexander MacKay and then by Sidney Orth in 1952. His pupils included Drs Rovenstine, Gillespie, Hingson, Lucien Morris, Gordh, Apgar (1909–75), Neff and many others.[24] Lived to enjoy 30 years of retirement, latterly growing citrus fruit in Florida, where he died in Orlando on 19 December 1979.

His contributions to the growing speciality were numerous and important and he wrote more than a hundred papers. Among the more noteworthy are the following: insistence on proper training programmes for young anaesthetists; encouragement on careful note-keeping during anaesthesia by means of punch-cards; the introduction of cyclopropane into anaesthetic practice;[25] the development of the to-and-fro carbon dioxide absorption system;[26] a re-evaluation of chloroform;[27] pioneering use of thiopentone in 1934[28] and endobronchial intubation.[29]

---

possibly even beneficial,[23] although this would not be the modern view.

Francis Hoeffer McMechan (1879–1939) (Figure 4.5) was an important figure in the development of societies of anaesthesia in the USA and in the English-speaking world.

Pioneers working on the pharmacodynamics of inhalation agents in the 1950s were S. S. Kety and E. Eger, who determined the rate at which the arterial partial pressure of an agent approached that of inspired gas.[24] The diffusion hypoxia that may occur on emergence from nitrous oxide anaesthesia was described by Fink.[31]

Specific inhalation agents

Many different anaesthetic agents have been tried. Lyman[39] describes those used in the first 30 years of anaesthesia. In the twentieth century many were described in successive editions of Hewer, C. L. *Recent Advances in Anaesthesia and Analgesia*, published in London by Churchill.

Ethylene

First prepared by Ingenhauss in 1779. Narcotic action is said to have been known to Simpson and to Nunelly in Leeds. Investigations were carried out in the USA by Luckhart, Carter, Easson Brown and others. The commercial gas was compressed in cylinders. The garlic-like smell was reminiscent of acetylene. It was more potent than nitrous oxide, had a shorter induction, and more oxygen could be used with it. Some salivary secretion occurred. The main disadvantage was that the gas was flammable (within limits of 3.05–28.5% in air, and 3.1–79.9% in oxygen). It was used mainly in the USA where 20 explosions were reported.[40]

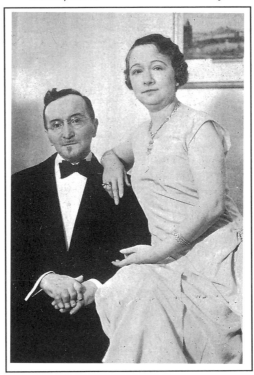

Figure 4.5   Francis Hoeffer McMechan (1879–1939)[80] and his wife Laurette

Started work as an anaesthetist in Cincinnati, but became afflicted with arthritis at an early age, and was soon unable to continue practice. Had married Laurette Van Varsevold, a descendant of Baron Larrey, whom he met when she was a student in the Cincinnati School of Acting, and who became a great support as he became immobilized, confined to a wheelchair, with restricted head and jaw movements and unable to feed himself. With the help of his wife, McMechan became interested in publications and the organization of societies.

The introductory number of the *American Journal of Surgery, Quarterly Supplement of Anesthesia and Analgesia*, which became the official organ of the American Association of Anesthetists and (for a time) of the Scottish Society of Anaesthetists, was published in 1914 with McMechan as Editor. Also edited the first series of *American Yearbooks of Anaesthesia and Analgesia* of which two volumes were published.

The Interstate Association of Anaesthetists held its first meeting in Cincinnati in 1915 with McMechan as Secretary. In 1920 the National Anesthesia Research Society was initiated. This soon became the International Anaesthesia Research Society with McMechan as Secretary-General. This met in 1922, the first number of *Current Researches in Anesthesia and Analgesia* being published in the same year with McMechan as Editor, a post he held until his death in 1939.

He was instrumental in the organization of regional societies of anaesthetists in many parts of the USA and Canada, and became known for his skill in the organization of meetings. Travelled extensively and could address audiences in French and German languages, and made many friends worldwide. His wife helped him overcome the physical difficulties of travelling and feeding. Visited England in 1928, Australia and New Zealand in 1929 where he was an inspiration to the young Geoffrey Kaye, and was instrumental in the foundation of the Australian Society of Anaesthetists. A visit to the continent of Europe failed to stimulate the formation of societies in the surgeon-dominated anaesthetic scene.

In 1937 he was not well enough to attend the 16th Annual Congress of Anesthetists, when a loving cup was presented to him. He died in 1939.

Acetylene

Known to produce anaesthesia in animals in 1895.[41] Used in Germany under the name Narcylen, and also in the USA. Characteristics were similar to those of ethylene, with rapid induction and recovery and the possibility of administering oxygen up to 50%.[42] It was flammable (2.8–50% in air, and 3–90% in oxygen). Explosions were reported.[43]

Other volatile agents

A number of volatile agents have enjoyed transient popularity. These include methyl-*n*-propyl ether, for which rapid smooth recovery with prolonged analgesia was claimed,[44] ethyl vinyl ether (Vinamar) whose use was first suggested by Leake and Chen in 1930[45] and was thought best used for light planes of anaesthesia,[46] and trifluoroethyl vinyl ether (Fluoromar).[47]

Xenon

First reported use as an anaesthetic agent was in 1951. Its potency was similar to ethylene, with minimal biochemical disturbances. It is non-flammable, but expensive to prepare. It has been used in studies of cerebral blood flow.[48]

Nitrous oxide

In 1956 H. C. A. Lassen, Copenhagen physician, reported that very prolonged nitrous oxide anaesthesia could cause bone-marrow aplasia.[49] Nitrous oxide interference with folate metabolism following prolonged inhalation was discovered in the 1960s.[50] Nitrous oxide was also found to inactivate the vitamin B_{12} component (cobalamin) of the enzyme methionine synthetase. The onset of inhibition was studied in the rodent,[51] but was thought to be much slower in man.[52] Falls of plasma methionine concentrations, requiring a period of at least 8 h of nitrous oxide anaesthesia, were noted in the late 1970s.[53]

Two cases of poisoning, one of which was fatal, in the UK due to impurities present in nitrous oxide were reported in detail by Clutton-Brock.[54] Investigation showed that a batch of nitrous oxide had become contaminated with the toxic substances nitric oxide (NO) and nitrogen dioxide (NO_2). The clinical features were cyanosis (methaemoglobinaemia), respiratory difficulty and circulatory failure, which could be delayed for several hours. A crude test for contamination with nitric oxide was developed.[55] It consisted of putting a piece of moistened starch iodide paper into a large syringe and then filling this with the test nitrous oxide mixed with 25% oxygen and waiting for 10 min. If the gas was contaminated by over 300 p.p.m., the starch iodide turned blue.

Premixed nitrous oxide and oxygen

Premixed nitrous oxide and oxygen (80:20) at a maximum cylinder pressure of 4700 kPa (700 lb/in²) was used in the USA in 1945.[56] Certain mixtures of nitrous oxide and oxygen were found to remain in the gaseous phase at pressures and temperatures (above −7°C) at which nitrous oxide by itself would normally be a liquid (Poynting effect). Entonox (50:50 mixture) was sold commercially.

Trichloroethylene

First described in 1864 by E. Fischer (1852–1919), chemist, of Jena,[57] since when it has been used in industry both as a fat solvent and in the dry-cleaning trade. Its poisonous properties have long been recognized,[58] especially its power to produce analgesia in distribution of the fifth cranial nerve and relieve trigeminal neuralgia. General anaesthetic effects described by Karl B. Lehmann (1858–1940) of Würzburg in 1911[59] and by Dennis Jackson[60] of Cincinnati in 1933. Cecil Striker[61] used it to anaesthetize 300 patients in 1935, but its introduction to European anaesthesia was due to Christopher Langton Hewer (1896–1986)* of St. Bartholomew's Hospital, London, who published case reports in 1941.[63]

---

* Christopher Langton Hewer (1896–1986)[62]

Qualified in medicine from St. Bartholomew's Hospital in 1918 and after a short period of service in the RAMC returned to St. Bartholomew's in 1919, being appointed to the staff as 'Administrator of Anaesthetics' at the early age of 24, working at that time with H. E. G. Boyle. Was an influential figure in the development of anaesthesia. Was Editor of *Anaesthesia* for 20 years from the foundation of the journal in 1946. Wrote the book *Anaesthesia for Children* in 1922 and was co-author with Boyle of *Practical Anaesthetics* in 1923, but is best known as author and later editor of *Recent Advances in Anaesthesia and Analgesia*, the first edition being published in 1932 and the 14th in 1982, before he retired – a span of 50 years. Was one of the 21 Foundation Fellows of the Faculty of Anaesthetists in 1948 and later became an examiner.

In his clinical work he placed emphasis on patient safety. Famous patients included royalty, Winston Churchill and George Bernard Shaw. Was largely responsible for the introduction of trichloroethylene as an alternative to the flammable ether and the potentially dangerous chloroform during World War II.

If used in a closed circuit with soda-lime, toxic products could be formed,[64] the most important being dichloracetylene. This is a potent nerve poison and produced temporary or permanent paralysis of cranial nerves or even death. The Vth and VIIth nerves were most commonly involved, and also the IIIrd, IVth, VIth, Xth and XIIth nerves. It was decomposed into phosgene ($COCl_2$) and hydrochloric acid at temperatures above 125°C during cautery, especially in the presence of oxygen.

Furthermore, induction was very slow. Cardiovascular stability was good, although dysrhythmias are seen, and the heart was sensitized to the effects of adrenaline. There was troublesome tachypnoea, though this could be controlled with opiates. Postoperative nausea and vomiting were common. It was, however, an excellent analgesic and was used in both surgery and in obstetrics.

Cyclopropane

Cyclopropane (trimethylene) was first synthesized by August von Freund (1835–92) of Poland[65] in 1882. Its anaesthetic properties were shown by G. W. H. Lucas and V. E. Henderson, of Toronto, in 1929,[66] and used on a human volunteer by W. Easson Brown, the patient being Professor Henderson.

It was stored in orange cylinders as a liquid at a pressure of 5 bar, no reducing valves being required. It was flammable and explosive. Its advantages were: very rapid induction, using 30–50% concentration in oxygen; and cardiac output was usually increased with arterial pressure well maintained, even in very ill patients. However, it was a powerful respiratory depressant, and vagotonic and ventricular dysrhythmias were seen, with some deaths from ventricular fibrillation. These complications were largely eliminated by controlled respiration (preventing hypercapnia). Nausea and vomiting were common postoperatively. Some anaesthetists found it useful in old, ill and shocked patients. It was also popular for induction in children until the 1980s.

Methoxyflurane

First used in clinical anaesthesia by Artusio and Van Poznak in 1960.[67] It had an unpleasant smell, was non-flammable, non-explosive, had no reaction with soda-lime, and was a good analgesic. However it had a very slow induction, and a significant amount was metabolized to fluoride, toxic to the kidneys. High output renal failure could follow.[68]

Halothane

The introduction of halothane into clinical practice in 1956 with calibrated vaporizers was a great step forward for anaesthesia. This introduced a phase of history in which the drug companies became the main originators of progress and development in the field of anaesthetic drugs. Halothane was synthesized in the laboratories of Imperial Chemical Industries near Manchester by C. W. Suckling in 1951,[69] and its pharmacology studied by James Raventós (1905–1983)[70] in succeeding years. Used clinically in 1956 by M. Johnstone[71] of Manchester followed by R. Bryce-Smith and H. D. O'Brien[72] of Oxford.

Enflurane

The first clinical account of enflurane appeared in 1966.[73] It was developed by Ross Terrell in the USA in 1963.

Isoflurane

Isoflurane is a fluorinated methyl ethyl ether originally synthesized by Ross Terrell in 1965. The same worker had synthesized its isomer, enflurane, in 1963.[74] Isoflurane was used in clinical anaesthesia by Dobkin and co-workers in 1971[75] and Stevens and co-workers[76] in the same year. This was followed by a messy accusation that it caused malignancies, eventually refuted by Eger. It has subsequently proved to be an enormous success, with few important side-effects.

Desflurane

This fluorinated methyl ethyl ether was developed in the USA.[77] In the UK it was first given to volunteers at Guy's Hospital.[78]

Sevoflurane

First used in North America in 1971.[79] The most extensive early experience was obtained in Japan.

References

1. Meyer, H.H. *Arch. Exp. Path. Pharmak.*, 1899, **42**, 109; Overton, C.E. *Studien über Narkose*. G. Fischer, Jena 1901. English translation by R. L. Lipnick, Chapman and Hall, London, 1990
2. Hewitt, F. *Lancet*, 1885, **1**, 840
3. McKesson, E.I. *Am. J. Surg. (Anesth. Suppl.)*, 1916, **7**, Feb., 415; Courville, C.B. *Medicine*, 1936, **15**, 129 (reprinted in 'Classical File', *Surv. Anesthesiol.*, 1958, **2**, 523, 660)
4. Wilson Smith, T. *Lancet*, 1898, **1**, 1005
5. Hewitt, F. *Lancet*, 1908, **1**, 490
6. Bloomfield, J. *Br. J. Anaesth.* 1926–7, **4**, 116–131
7. See Edwards, G. *Ann. R. Coll. Surg.*, 1951, **8**, 233
8. Binning, R. *Anaesthesia*, 1978, **33**, 55
9. Crile, G.W. *Lancet*, 1913, **2**, 7; *Surg. Gynecol. Obstet.*, 1911, **13**, 170; *Ann. Surg.*, 1908, **47**, 866; *Boston Med. Surg. J.*, 1910, **10**, 291
10. Lundy, J.S. *Minnesota Med.*, 1926, **9**, 399 (reprinted in 'Classical File', *Surv. Anesthesiol.*, 1981, **25**, 272)
11. Rees, G.J. and Gray, T.C. *Br. J. Anaesth.*, 1950, **22**, 83; Boulton, T.B. *Surv. Anesthesiol.*, 1994, **38**, 239–252
12. Gray, T.C. *Ir. J. Med. Sci.* 1960, **419**, 499
13. Condon, H.A. and Gilchrist, E. *Anaesthesia*, 1986, **41**, 46–52; Boulton, T.B. Sir Ivan Magill and anaesthesia for thoracic surgery. *Surv. Anesthesiol.* 'Classical File', 1988, **32**, 387–398; Bamji, A. *Curr. Anaesth. Crit. Care*, 1996, in press
14. Macintosh, R.R. (1897–1989) In J. Rupreht *et al.* (eds.) *Anaesthesia; Essays on its History*, Springer-Verlag, Berlin, 1985, p.352; Boulton, T.B. Professor Sir Robert Macintosh: personal reflections on a remarkable man and his career. *Regional Anaesthesia*, 1993, **18**, 149–154
15. Haldane, J.S. *Br. Med. J.*, 1917, **1**, 181
16. O'Sullivan, J. *Br. J. Pharmaceut. Pract.*, 1988, **10**, 395
17. Herman, L. and Escher, T. *Pflügers Arch. Ges. Physiol.*, 1870, **3**, 3
18. Henderson, Y. *Br. Med. J.*, 1925, **2**, 1170
19. Razis, P. *Anaesthesia*, 1989, **44**, 348
20. Waters, R.M., *Curr. Res. Anesth. Analg.*, 1924, **3**, 20; Waters, R.M. *et al. Curr. Res. Anesth. Analg.* 1931, **10**, 10
21. Jackson, D.E. *J. Lab. Clin. Med.*, 1915, **1**, 1
22. Leake, C.D. and Waters, R.M., *Anesth. Analg. Curr. Res.*, 1929, **8**, 17
23. Geddes, I.C. and Gray, T.C. *Lancet*, 1959, 24
24. Morris, L.E. In *Anaesthesia; Essays on its History*, edited by J. Rupreht *et al.*, Springer-Verlag, Berlin, 1985, p.32; Gordh, T. *ibid.* p.36
25. Stiles, J.A. *et al. Curr. Res. Anesth. Analg.*, 1934, **13**, 56
26. Waters, R.M. *Curr. Res. Anesth. Analg.*, 1924, **3**, 20
27. Waters, R.M. (ed.) *Chloroform: A Study after 100 Years*, University of Wisconsin Press, Madison, 1951
28. Pratt, T.W. *et al. Am. J. Surg.*, 1936, **31**, 464
29. Gale, J.W. and Waters, R.M. *J. Thorac. Surg.*, 1932, **1**, 432
30. Kety, S.S. *Anesthesiology*, 1950, **11**, 517; Eger, E.J. *Anesthetic Uptake and Action*, Williams and Wilkins, Baltimore, 1974

31. Fink, B.R. *Anesthesiology*, 1955, **16**, 511; Fink, B.R. *et al. Fed. Proc.*, 1954, **13**, 354
32. See also Waters, R.M. Eminent anaesthetists: A. E. Guedel. *Br. J. Anaesth.*, 1952, **24**, 292; Neff, W.B. In *The Genesis of Contemporary American Anesthesiology*, edited by P. P. Volpitto and L. D. Vandam, Thomas, Springfield Ill., 1961; Calverley, R. K. In *Anaesthesia; Essays on its History*, edited by J. Rupreht *et al.*, Springer-Verlag, Berlin, 1985, p.18
33. Reprinted in 'Classical File', *Surv. Anesthesiol.*, 1979, **23**, 340
34. Guedel, A.E. and Waters, R.M. *Curr. Res. Anesth. Analg.*, 1928, **7**, 238
35. *Curr. Res. Anesth.*, 1920, **1**, 26; *Inhalation Anesthesia, A Fundamental Guide*, Macmillan, New York, 1937
36. Guedel, A.E. (1933) *J.A.M.A.*, 1933, **103**, 1862
37. *Curr. Res. Anesth. Analg.*, 1934, **13**, 116
38. *Anesthesiology*, 1940, **1**, 1
39. Lyman, H.M. *Artificial Anaesthesia and Anaesthetics*, Appleton, New York, 1880
40. Herb, I.C. *J. Am. Med. Assoc.*, 1933, 25 Nov., 1716
41. Roseman, R. *Arch. Exp. Path. Pharm.*, 1895, **36**, 179
42. Goldman, A. and Goldman J.P. *Br. J. Anaesth.*, 1924, **2**, 122
43. Hurler, K. *Munch. Med. Woch.*, 1924, **71**, 1432
44. Barnett, M.S. *Anaesthesia*, 1954, **9**, 153
45. Leake, C.D. and Chen, M.Y. *Proc. Soc. Exp. Biol.*, 1930, **28**, 151
46. Dornette, W.H.L. and Orth, O.S. *Anesth. Analg.*, 1955, **34**, 26
47. Orth, O.S. *Fed. Proc.*, 1955, **14**, 376; Sadove, M.S. *et al. Anesthesiology*, 1956, **17**, 591; Gainza, E., Heaton, C.E., Willcox, M. and Virtue, R.W. *Br. J. Anaesth.*, 1956, **28**, 411
48. Cullen, S.C. and Gross, E.G. *Fed. Proc.*, 1951, **10**, 290; Fink, B.R. *Anesthesiology*, 1955, **16**, 511
49. Lassen, H.C.A. *Lancet*, 1956, **1**, 525
50. Bank, R.G.S. and Henderson, R.J. *J. Chem. Soc. (A)*, 1968, **28**, 86
51. Deacon, R. *et al. Eur. J. Biochem.*, 1980, **104**, 419; Koblin, D.D. *et al. Anesthesiology*, 1981, **54**, 318
52. Koblin, D.D. *et al. Anesth. Analg.*, 1982, **61**, 75
53. Amess, J.A.L. *et al. Lancet*, 1978, **2**, 339; Amos, R.J. *et al. Lancet*, 1982, **2**, 835; Nunn, J.F. *et al. Br. J. Anaesth.*, 1986, **58**, 1
54. Clutton-Brock, J. *Br. J. Anaesth.*, 1967, **39**, 343, 388; Editorial. *Lancet*, 1967, **2**, 930
55. Kain, M.L. *et al. Br. J. Anaesth.*, 1967, **39**, 425
56. Barach, A.L. and Rovenstine, E.A. *Anesthesiology*, 1945, **6**, 449
57. Fischer, E. *Jena Z. Med. Naturw.*, 1864, **1**, 123
58. Plessner, W. *Berl. Klin. Wochenschr.*, 1916, **53**, 25
59. Lehmann, K.B. *Arch. Hyg. Berl.*, 1911, **74**, 1
60. Jackson, D.E. *Curr. Res. Anesth. Analg.*, 1934, **13**, 198
61. Striker, C. *et al. Curr. Res. Anesth. Analg.*, 1935, **14**, 68
62. See also Hewer, C.L. Forty years on (Frederick Hewitt Lecture). *Anaesthesia*, 1959, **14**, 311; Fifty years on. In *Recent Advances in Anaesthesia and Analgesia*, edited by R. S. Atkinson and C. L. Hewer,

Churchill Livingstone, Edinburgh, 1982; Boulton, T.B. *Anaesthesia*, 1986, **41**, 469

63. Hewer, C.L. and Hadfield, C.F. *Br. Med. J.*, 1941, **1**, 924 (reprinted in 'Classical File', *Surv. Anesthesiol.*, 1963, **7**, 924); Hewer, C.L. *Proc. Roy. Soc. Med.*, 1942, **35**, 463
64. Morton, H.J.V. *Br. Med. J.*, 1943, **2**, 838; McAuley, J. *Br. Med. J.* 1943, **2**, 713.
65. von Freund, A. *Monats. f. Chemie*, 1882, **3**, 625
66. Lucas, G.W.H. and Henderson, V.E. *Can. Med. Assoc. J.*, 1929, **21**, 173
67. Artusio, J.F. *et al. Anesthesiology*, 1960, **21**, 512 (reprinted in 'Classical File', *Surv. Anesthesiol.*, 1968, **12**, 196)
68. Paddock, R.B. *et al. Anaesthesiology*, 1964, **25**, 707; Cransell, W.B. *et al. Anaesthesiology*, 1966, **27**, 591; Richey, J.E. and Smith, R.B. *Anaesthesia*, 1972, **27**, 9
69. Suckling, C.W. *Br. J. Anaesth.*, 1957, **29**, 466
70. Raventós, J. *Br. J. Pharmacol.*, 1956, **11**, 394 (reprinted in 'Classical File', *Surv. Anesthesiol.*, 1966, **10**, 183)
71. Johnstone, M. *Br. J. Anaesth.*, 1956, **28**, 392
72. Bryce-Smith, R. and O'Brien, H.D. *Br. Med. J.*, 1956, **2**, 969; *Proc. Roy. Soc. Med.*, 1957, **30**, 193
73. Virtue, R.W. *et al. Can. Anaesth. Soc. J.*, 1966, **12**, 233 (reprinted in 'Classical File', *Surv. Anesthesiol.*, 1977, **21**, 210)
74. Vircha, J.F. *Anesthesiology*, 1971, **21**, 4
75. Dobkin, A.B. *et al. Can. Anaesth. Soc. J.*, 1971, **18**, 264
76. Stevens, D.J. *et al. Can. Anaesth. Soc. J.*, 1971, **18**, 500
77. Eger, E.I. *Anesth. Analg.*, 1987, **66**, 983
78. Jones, R.M. *et al. Br. J. Anaesth.*, 1990, **64**, 11
79. Wallin, R.F. and Napoli, M.D. *Fed. Proc.*, 1971, **30**, 442
80. Waters, R.M. *J. Hist. Med. Allied Sci.*, 1946, **1**, 595–606; Wilson, G. *Fifty Years On, The Australian Society of Anaesthetists 1934–1984*, Australian Society of Anaesthetists, Edgecliff, NSW, 1987.

5
Anaesthetic apparatus

For a full discussion of this important subject, see the book by K. Bryn Thomas, *The Development of Anaesthetic Apparatus*, Blackwell, Oxford, 1975. The development of standards in the evolution of anaesthetic equipment has been reviewed by Rendell-Baker.[1]

Open drop administration and simple inhalational apparatus

Earliest administrations of ether were through simple inhalers, e.g. as used by Morton (1846), Squire (1846), Charrière (1847), Dieffenbach (1847). A breathing tube was placed in the patient's mouth, and valves were normally used to separate inspired and expired air.

The open drop method of administration was introduced by Sir James Y. Simpson for chloroform in 1847, using a folded handkerchief. The advantages were cheapness, portability, ease of administration and minimal dead space. The disadvantages were uneven anaesthesia due to variations in concentration of vapour, risk of fire (except with chloroform), wastefulness, pollution of atmosphere, risk of damage to eyes or skin of patient from anaesthetic liquid and fall in oxygen concentration under the mask (which could be remedied by giving oxygen under the mask via a small catheter).

In the first 80 years of general anaesthesia, many millions of patients were managed satisfactorily using open masks. In the 1850s a 'common towel' was used by Syme and Lister[2] for chloroform drop administration. In 1862 Thomas Skinner, Liverpool general practitioner and obstetrician, invented a wire-frame mask, covered with domette,[3] and carried in the top hat.[4] This was copied by John Murray,[5] and by Friedrich von Esmarch, a German military surgeon, whose clip enabled the mask to be strapped to the face.[6] These masks gained wide acceptance.[7] Kirchhof added a trough-shaped

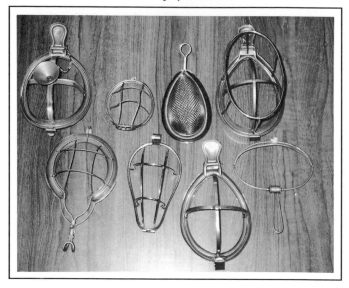

Figure 5.1 Schimmelbusch and other masks

rim to prevent liquid dropping on to the patient's skin, developed by Curt Schimmelbusch (1860–1895), Berlin surgeon and pioneer of aseptic surgery, in 1890 (Figure 5.1).[8] It could be used for ether or chloroform. G. H. Bellamy Gardner[9] of Charing Cross Hospital was a leading British exponent of the method (Figure 5.2).

What are now called anaesthetic masks, and were originally called face-pieces, were invented by Cloquet[10], and by Francis Sibson, Resident Surgical Officer at Nottingham General Hospital[11] in February 1847, as a development of the original mouth-tubes. Sibson's mask, made of mackintosh and lined with oiled silk, was improved by Snow, whose version was made of thin sheet-lead, covered with leather outside and velveteen inside, and fitted with valves to go with his newly-invented ether inhaler (see below).[12] Nasal masks were used instead of the face-piece mask for dental anaesthesia. Sibson's face-piece was capable of this.

In 1859 Fauré of Paris gave chloroform vapour through a rubber tube inserted in one nostril[13] for oral surgery, in much the same way that Malgaigne had given ether for the first time in France, in Paris in 1847. In 1861 A. E. Sansom repeated Fauré's work '... for prolonging anaesthesia ... in operations on the mouth'.[14] Alfred Coleman adapted Snow's chloroform inhaler in 1862 with a flattened silver tube with two tubular prongs for nasal inhalation, and

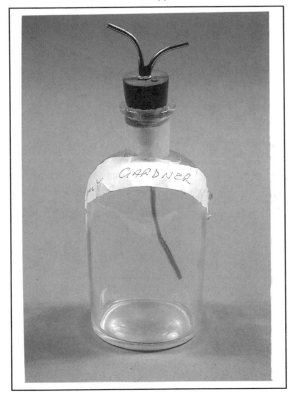

Figure 5.2　Bellamy Gardner dropper bottle

later a small nasal mask.[15] In the twentieth century they were further developed by McKesson and also Victor Goldman of London.

Anaesthetic machines[16]

Dates of introduction of some machines and their designers are as follows: Frederick Hewitt, 1898; Charles Teter of Cleveland, 1902; Karl Connell (1873–1941) New York anaesthetist, 1908; Elmer Isaac McKesson (1881–1935) of Toledo, Ohio, physiologist, anaesthetist and manufacturer, 1910; Walter R. Boothby (1880–1953) of the Mayo Clinic, 1912; Frederick J. Cotton (1869–1938) of Boston, 1912; James Tayloe Gwathmey (1863–1944) of New York, 1912; Richard von

Forregger (1873–1960), New York manufacturer, 1914; Henry Edmund Gaskin Boyle (1875–1941) London anaesthetist, 1917.*

Intermittent flow machines

Anaesthetic machines provided either continuous or intermittent flow of gas. The intermittent flow machines were either powered by gas pressure triggered by the patient ('demand' apparatus), or the flow was generated entirely by the patient's inspiration ('draw-over' apparatus). Demand apparatus was designed primarily for dental anaesthesia or for obstetric analgesia. Sir Frederic Hewitt designed the first practical apparatus in 1887 for giving oxygen and nitrous oxide mixtures,[18] in which reservoirs of the two gases mixed in a variable proportion at the face-piece, but the reservoirs were not pressurized.

The best-known true demand flow machine was devised by E. I. McKesson (1881–1935),† described in 1926,[19] and is still in use in

---

* Henry Edmund Gaskin Boyle (1875–1941)[17]

Born in Barbados and qualified at St. Bartholomew's Hospital, London, in 1901, where as a student he was president of the Abernethian Society. Became casualty officer in Bristol and then returned to St Bartholomew's as junior resident anaesthetist, rising in due course to become head of the department. About 1912, became interested in nitrous oxide and oxygen anaesthesia and in 1917 got Coxeter, the instrument maker, to copy James Tayloe Gwathmey's (1855–1943) gas and oxygen machine which became the first Boyle apparatus. It had water-sight flowmeters and his metal-and-glass ether vaporizer (Boyle's bottle). Introduced gas and oxygen into France for use in anaesthetizing wounded soldiers in World War I and for this received the decoration of OBE. After the war he visited the USA and brought back with him Davis's gag (G. Davis was anaesthetist to Harvey Cushing at the Johns Hopkins Hospital), which he introduced to British throat surgeons. He was an early user of Magill's endotracheal techniques and was elected FRCS and DA in 1935. Was one of the original pair of examiners for the latter diploma. A founder member of the Association of Anaesthetists of Great Britain and Ireland in 1932. In 1907 he wrote the first edition of his textbook *Practical Anaesthetics*, the third edition of which was prepared by his junior colleague C. Langton Hewer. Boyle was a character and was universally known as 'Cockie'.

† Elmer I. McKesson (1881–1935)

Born in Walkerton, Indiana, and graduated from Rush Medical School. Served as an intern in Toledo, and started his interest in anaesthesia there. His innovation led to the invention of many varied pieces of apparatus apart from the nitrous oxide and oxygen intermittent flow machine. He designed valves for demand gas flow, oxygen tents and machines for suction which were all manufactured by a local company in Toledo. Helped found the University of Toledo, and served as Professor of Physiology and Physiologic Chemistry.

some centres. It gave nitrous oxide and oxygen for dental anaesthesia, but could also be used as a continuous flow machine and could take a vaporizer for ether, or later for halothane. The Walton Five was a similar machine. R. J. Minnitt (1890–1974) of Liverpool designed the first demand flow machine for the self-administration of nitrous oxide and air during labour.[20]

Continuous flow machines

The best-known continuous flow machine was Henry Boyle's modification[21] of the American Gwathmey apparatus.[22] Another modification of Gwathmey's apparatus at that time was that of Marshall in London. One of Boyle's most important modifications was the addition of reducing valves. In the typical Boyle machine today, gases are delivered from cylinders or pipelines, each via a reducing valve which reduces the pressure to the needle valve flowmeters. Two or more vaporizers are usually provided and increasing amounts of the gases can be diverted through them. Gases then pass into a suitable breathing circuit.

The original Boyle machine of 1917 was built by the firm Coxeters, under the personal direction of Lord George Wellesley (a great-grandson of the first Duke of Wellington). In its original form it housed two nitrous oxide and two oxygen cylinders in a wooden box and used a water-sight flowmeter and an ether vaporizer. It had a pressure gauge on the oxygen cylinders, fine-adjustment reducing valves and a spirit flame to warm these and prevent obstruction of gas flow from freezing of water vapour, an impurity in early gas supplies. A Cattlin bag, a three-way stopcock and a face-mask completed the apparatus. A portable form was designed for use with the British Army in France, which both popularized it and familiarized a generation of service anaesthetists with its use. Once again, a world war was instrumental in the development of new techniques of anaesthesia. The modern Boyle's apparatus thus bears little resemblance to the original model (Figure 5.3), as subsequent modifications included:

- 1920 Addition of Boyle's vaporizing bottle to flowmeters
- 1926 Addition of second vaporizing bottle and bypass controls
- 1927 Addition of third water-sight feed tube for carbon dioxide
- 1930 Addition of plunger device to Boyle's bottle
- 1933 Dry bobbin type of flowmeter displaced the water-sight meter
- 1937 Rotameters displaced dry bobbin flowmeters
- 1952 Introduction of pin index system.

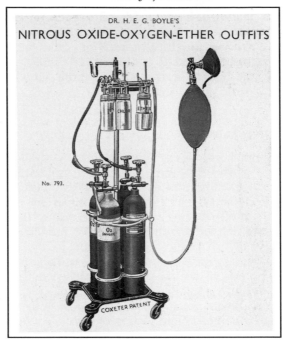

Figure 5.3   Early Boyle machine

Flowmeters

The rotameter was patented in Germany in 1908 by Karl Küppers of Aachen, and used in anaesthesia by Maximilian Neu,[23] an obstetrician and gynaecologist of Heidelberg, in 1910. Magill suggested its use independently in 1932 and used it a few years later. R. Salt developed it further in 1937.

Other devices to measure gas flow have included:

- Water-sight meter. The gases were passed through a perforated tube placed vertically in the liquid volatile agent, and the flow estimated from how many of the holes were generating bubbles. Used in the original Boyle's machine.
- The Heidbrink meter. A black inverted float, free to rise within a metal tube with a varying taper. The upper end projected into a glass tube, where the calibrations were visible.
- Connell meter. A pair of stainless steel balls moving within a tapered glass tube on an inclined plane.
- Pressure gauge meter. Measured the pressure drop across a fixed orifice, either with a Bourdon gauge or with a simple water

depression manometer (as in the Foregger flowmeter). This allowed easy measurement of low flows appropriate to closed circuit anaesthesia.

Vaporizers

The great unknown quantity of very early anaesthesia was the inhaled concentration of volatile agent. Clearly, safety would always be precarious until this could be controlled. There have been many attempts to do so, and just a few can be included here:

1847 John Snow's ether inhaler attempted to regulate the concentration of ether by controlling its temperature by placing a vaporizing chamber in a water bath held in a copper box. This was the first such attempt to do so. Snow adapted this in 1848 for use with chloroform.

1862 Joseph Clover designed a large bag to sling over his shoulder, which he would prefill with a known (4.5%) concentration of chloroform. This rendered a vaporizer unnecessary, but at the expense of being rather cumbersome.

1867 Junker's inhaler (F. A. Junker 1828–1901),[24] using air blown over chloroform with a hand pump, was an early example of a plenum-type vaporizer.

1903 Vernon Harcourt (1834–1919), physical chemist at Oxford University, designed an inhaler to limit the concentration of chloroform (in air) to about 2%.[25]

1908 Louis Ombrédanne (1871–1956), Paris surgeon, described his ether–air inhaler.

1916 Sir F. E. Shipway (1875–1968) of Guy's Hospital, London, introduced his apparatus[26] for insufflating warm ether vapour.

1940 The Oxford vaporizer[27] was developed by Robert Macintosh in collaboration with Morris Motors for use by the Armed Forces in 1940–41. Transfer of heat from a water jacket was facilitated by the latent heat of crystallization of calcium chloride. A total of 1700 were distributed to the Armed Forces anaesthetists during World War II. A chloroform version was designed for use by airborne units (flammable ether was not allowed on aeroplanes or on parachute descents). Further drawover units are described below.

The introduction of halothane as a potent volatile agent required suitably accurate and reliable vaporizers. The tec series ('*temperature compensated*') proved very popular, and have been adapted for all other current volatile agents. That for desflurane, with its extreme volatility, has been heated and pressurized.

Another approach to the vaporization of volatile agents was the supply of a saturated vapour which could then be diluted according to requirements. This was particularly appropriate when the agent had to be introduced via the low gas flow needed for closed circuits. In 1921 the Pinson bomb was an apparatus whereby ether in a rigid container was immersed in warm water so that the ether was vaporized; the whole apparatus was analogous to a gas cylinder which delivered ether as a vapour.[28]

A much later vaporizer was the Copper Kettle[29] which supplied a saturated vapour, the use of copper in the apparatus being to facilitate heat transfer to the liquid ether and minimize the fall in concentration of the ether. The principle was then transferred to the use of halothane and other inhalation agents. In Britain, a variation was the Halox vaporizer, made of glass with a compensation mechanism to allow for temperature changes. Goldman, McKesson and Rowbotham all introduced low-resistance vaporizers designed for halothane use in a demand breathing system. They were all similar, and were not accurately calibrated or compensated for changes in temperature.

Draw-over apparatus

This equipment was developed especially for 'field' use where nitrous oxide was not available and where portability was important. For example, the Flagg can[30] was devised during World War I. The patient breathed to and fro through a can containing ether. It was improvised from available material (e.g. coffee jar, food tins) and control over vapour strength was achieved by admitting air as a diluent.[31]

The best-known draw-over apparatus is probably the EMO inhaler (Epstein–Macintosh–Oxford) (Figure 5.4).[32] It was fairly bulky (24 × 23cm) and weighed 6.5 kg when the water compartment was full. It was developed from the original wartime Oxford vaporizer in the Nuffield Department of Anaesthetics in the University of Oxford. It delivered a predetermined concentration of ether vapour in air, the accuracy of which was greatest at high concentrations and high tidal volumes.[33] It was only suitable for plenum use (continuous flow) if the carrier gas was greater than 10 l/min.[34] It had an automatic thermocompensator bellows mechanism. A water compartment of approximately 1200 ml acted as a heat buffer. It could be combined with an Oxford inflating bellows[35] for intermittent positive pressure ventilation (IPPV).

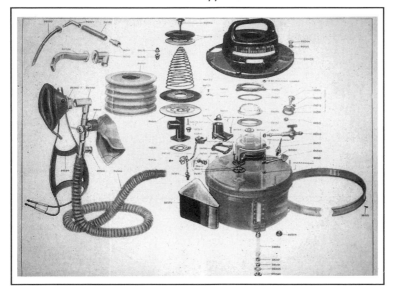

Figure 5.4   Exploded view of the EMO inhaler

The Oxford Miniature Vaporizer[36] was originally developed as an induction unit. This had a water jacket, and could be calibrated for halothane, trichloroethylene, chloroform and methoxyflurane. It was used (with halothane) to smooth induction with the EMO ether inhaler, and – with the Oxford inflating bellows – for IPPV. Two of these vaporizers (for trichloroethylene and halothane) were incorporated into the Triservice anaesthetic apparatus which remains in military use. Other portable anaesthetic machines, e.g. Portablease and Fluoxair, used a low-resistance draw-over vaporizer and an inflating bellows with one-way valves and facilities for oxygen enrichment.[37]

Gas delivery systems (breathing circuits)

Semi-closed systems

The different systems, combinations of breathing tubes, expiratory valves, masks and reservoir bags, designed so as to prevent the rebreathing of alveolar gas, were classified in 1954 by W. W. Mapleson, the physicist, in Cardiff.[38] The Mapleson 'A' circuit is also called the Magill circuit or attachment.[39] Coaxial versions have been described for convenience and are in common use, e.g. Bain's version (1972) of the Mapleson 'D',[40] and Lack's version (1976) of

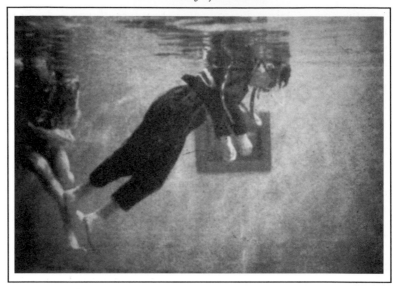

Figure 5.5   An unconscious E. A. Pask in water

the Mapleson 'A'.[41] The principle of the Mapleson 'D' circuit was first used by R. R. Macintosh and E. A. Pask during World War II for experiments on the buoyant qualities of life-jackets (the Mae West) worn by unconscious subjects.[42] The late E. A. Pask very staunchly allowed himself to be anaesthetized with ether on many occasions (Figure 5.5), during these experiments, and gave his name to the Pask Medal of the Association of Anaesthetists of Great Britain and Ireland.

The Mapleson 'E' circuit is Ayre's T-piece, developed for paediatric use as it contained no valves and was small and light.[43] It was further modified by addition of a 500 ml bag into the familiar Jackson Rees configuration, to allow respiratory monitoring and the use of ventilation by hand.[44]

Rebreathing systems with carbon dioxide absorption

A rebreathing system was originally used by John Snow in 1850,[45] who demonstrated on himself that anaesthesia was prolonged by rebreathing the chloroform present in expired air. He also used the apparatus, which contained caustic potash, to measure the production of carbon dioxide during anaesthesia, and found it to be less than he had expected, showing the depressant effect of anaesthesia on metabolism. Carbon dioxide absorption was also used by Franz Kuhn (1866–1929), of Kassel, in 1906 in Germany.[46]

Such systems had other uses. A closed circuit system for use by coalminers was described by Theodore Schwann (1810–82), known for his nerve cells, and professor in the University of Liege, in 1877.[47] The systems were revised by Dennis Jackson (1878–1930) of Cincinnati in 1915 for work on animals (after working on problems of ventilation in submarines during World War I),[48] and by Waters in 1920 for clinical anaesthesia.[49] The threat of gas warfare from 1914 to 1918 had improved the ways of manufacturing soda lime to increase its efficiency.

In the Waters 'to-and-fro' system,[50] gases passed through a canister of soda lime during both inspiration and expiration. Fresh gases were led to the patient close to the mask. The circle system was devised by Brian Sword (1889–1956) of North Carolina[51] in 1926. W. B. Primrose (1892–1977), of Glasgow, used caustic soda solution as an absorber in 1931,[52] while Dräger had patented an apparatus with a closed system in 1926.[53]

Tracheal insufflation via a small catheter used by Elsberg of New York in 1909 and by Magill and C. Langton Hewer of London[54] was the forerunner of endotracheal anaesthesia, which is discussed in Chapter 9.

Ventilators[55]

The concept of artificial ventilation can be said to go back to the Old Testament: ' . . . then the Lord God formed man of dust from the ground, and breathed into his nostrils the breath of life; and man became a living being' (*Genesis* 2:7) or, more scientifically, to the demonstration by Vesalius in 1543 that blowing intermittently down a reed passed into the trachea of an animal could maintain life. Hooke performed this experiment on a dog in 1667 using a tracheotomy and bellows as a ventilator.[56]

Two developments stimulated the creation of early ventilators: advances in resuscitation in the nineteenth century, and the need to avoid the problems of the open pneumothorax during thoracic surgery (see Chapters 9, 12 and 18). Northrup was probably the first, in 1896, to report the use of the Fell–O'Dwyer apparatus of an endotracheal tube and bellows in the ventilatory support of eight patients. The four who had opium poisoning all survived.[57] The American surgeon Matas was a pioneer in the use of this apparatus for thoracotomy, developing bellows operated by a piston and motor.[58]

Yet IPPV was not generally exploited for surgery in the early 1900s in the way that it was in experimental physiological laboratories. Possibly the surgeons were wary of a technique that depended much on the skills of others. Indeed, considerable effort was put into negative pressure ventilators for surgery, as with Sauerbruch's chamber which contained the body of the patient and the surgeon(s), with the patient's head and the anaesthetist outside. Breathing was generated by intermittent negative chamber pressure of 7 mmHg.[59]

There was a similar development of negative pressure 'tank' ventilators for patients with diseases such as poliomyelitis. These had been conceived as early as 1832,[60] but the significant landmarks were Thunberg's Barospirator,[61] (1924) in which the whole body was enclosed, and the modification by Shaw and Drinker in 1929,[62] in which the head was left outside and a collar formed a gas-tight seal, was a much more effective arrangement. This 'iron lung' became the main treatment for paralytic polio until the 1950s.

There were a few pioneers of positive pressure ventilation before the introduction of relaxants, and one of the best known was Crafoord in Sweden in 1940. He used Frenckner's Spiropulsator[63] which had been developed at the suggestion of the Swedish surgeon Giertz, a former assistant to Sauerbruch. The use of curare naturally made such techniques much easier. Trier Mørch (then of Copenhagen) designed his own version of the Spiropulsator in 1947.[64] Other early ventilators were by Pinson,[65] Blease[66] and Engström.[67] The latter became especially popular for intensive care.

The polio epidemics of the 1950s demonstrated the need for versatile and powerful ventilators, and happily the advantages of such techniques in many branches of surgery became well established. At the same time, technology provided the means to construct increasingly reliable machines, and to monitor the patient, especially by arterial blood gas analysis. Today we have available a profusion of electrically- and gas-powered ventilators with integral monitoring devices.

References

1. Rendell-Baker, J. In *Anaesthesia: Essays on its History,* edited by J. Rupreht and M. I. van Lieburg, Springer-Verlag, Berlin, 1985, p.159
2. *The Collected Papers of Joseph, Baron Lister,* Vol. 1, Oxford, 1909, pp.140, 143
3. *Retrosp. Pract. Med.,* 1862, **46,** 185
4. Correspondence, *Br. Med. J.,* 1873, **1,** 353
5. *Br. Med. J.,* 1868, **1,** 535
6. Esmarch, F. *Chirurgie de Guerre,* 1879, Paris, pp.112, 113
7. Kappeler, O. *Anaesthetica Deutsche Chirurgie,* 1880, **20,** 144

8. Schimmelbusch, C. *Ill. Mschr. Arztl. Polyt.*, 1890, **12**, 203; *Index Medicus*, 1890, **12**, 615; *Anleitung Z. aseptischen Wundbehandling*, Hirschwald, Berlin, 1894
9. Bellamy Gardner, G. H. *Br. Med. J.*, 1907, **2**, 1516; *Br. Med. J.*, 1910, **2**, 766
10. *Bull. Acad. Med. Paris*, 1846–7, **12**, 348
11. Sibson, F. *Lond. Med. Gaz.*, 1847, **4**, 363
12. Snow, J. *On the inhalation of the vapour of ether in surgical operations*, London, 1847, p.22
13. *Arch. Gén. Méd.*, 1859, **1**, 633; *Bull. Acad. Méd. Paris*, 1859–60, **25**, 115
14. *Med. Times, Lond.*, 1861, **1**, 550
15. Coleman, A. *Manual of Dental Surgery*, 1888, pp.275, 276
16. Thompson, P.W. and Wilkinson, D.J. *Br. J. Anaesth.*, 1985, **57**, 640; Rendell-Baker, L. and Pettis, J.L. *The History of Anaesthesia*, edited by R. S. Atkinson and T. B. Boulton, RSM, London, 1989, pp.402–425
17. Wilkinson, D.J., *Curr. Anaesth. Crit. Care*, 1996, in press
18. Hewitt, F.W. *Anaesthetics and their Administration*, Griffin, London, 1893; *The Administration of Nitrous Oxide and Oxygen for Dental Operations*, Ash, London, 1897
19. McKesson, E.I. *Br. Med. J.*, 1926, **2**, 1113
20. Minnitt, R.J. (1950) *Proc. Roy. Soc. Med.*, 1934, **27**, 1313
21. Boyle, H.E.G. *Br. Med. J.*, 1917, **2**, 653; Hadfield, C.F. (1950) Eminent anaesthetists: H. E. G. Boyle, *Br. J. Anaesth.*, 1950, **22**, 107; Hewer, C. Langton, *Anaesthesia* 1967, **22**, 357; Obituary of Boyle, *Anaesthesia*, 1967, **22**, 710; Watt, O. M. *Anaesthesia*, 1968, **23**, 103; Bryn Thomas, K. (1975) *The Development of Anaesthetic Apparatus*, Blackwell, Oxford, 1975, p.144; Hewer, C.L. *Anaesthesia*, 1977, **32**, 908
22. Gwathmey, J. T. *Anesthesia*, Appleton, New York, 1914, p.174
23. Neu, M., *Münch. Med. Wochenschr.*, 1910, **57**, 1873
24. *Med. Times & Gaz.*, 1867, **2**, 590; *ibid.*, 1868, **1**, 171; Boulton T. B. (1985) Origins of the plenum principle of vaporization. *Surv. Anesthesiol.* 'Classical File', 1985, **29**, 201–206
25. Harcourt, V. *Br. Med. J.* 18 July 1903
26. Shipway, F. E. *Lancet* 1916, **1**, 70
27. Beinart, J. *A History of the Nuffield Department of Anaesthetics, Oxford 1937–1987*, Oxford Medical Publications, 1987, p.54
28. Wilson, S. R. and Pinson, K. B. A warm ether bomb. *Lancet*, 1921, **1**, 336
29. Morris L. A. New vaporiser for liquid anesthetics. *Anesthesiology*, 1952, **13**, 587
30. Flagg, P. J. *The Art of Anaesthesia*, 7th edn, Lippincott, Philadelphia, 1954
31. Boulton, T. B. *Anaesthesia*, 1966, **21**, 513
32. Epstein, H. G. and Macintosh, R. R. *Anaesthesia*, 1956, **11**, 83
33. Marsh, D. R. G. and Herbert, P. *Anaesthesia*, 1983, **38**, 575
34. Schaefer, H.-G. and Farman, J. V. *Anaesthesia*, 1984, **39**, 171
35. Macintosh, R. R. *Br. Med. J.*, 1953, **2**, 202
36. Parkhouse, J. *Anaesthesia*, 1966, **21**, 498
37. Merrifield, A. J. *et al. Br. J. Anaesth.*, 1967, **39**, 50

38. Mapleson, W. W. *Br. J. Anaesth.*, 1954, **26**, 323
39. Magill, I. W. *Proc. Roy. Soc. Med.*, 1929, **22**, 83; 1967, *ibid.*, **60**, 16
40. Bain, J. A. and Spoerel, W. E. *Can. Anaesth. Soc. J.*, 1972, **19**, 426
41. Lack, J. A. *Anaesthesia*, 1976, **31**, 259, 576
42. Macintosh, R. R. and Mushin, W. W. *Med. Times*, 1945, **73**, 53; Macintosh, R. R. and Pask, E. A. *Br. J. Indust. Med.*, 1957, **14**, 168
43. Ayre, T. P. *Lancet*, 1937, **1**, 561; *Curr. Res. Anesth. Analg.*, 1937, **16**, 330; *Br. J. Surg.*, 1937, **35**, 131 (reprinted in 'Classical File', *Surv. Anesthesiol.*, 1967, **11**, 400); *Br. J. Anaesth.*, 1956, **28**, 520; *Anaesthesia*, 1967, **22**, 359
44. Rees, G. J. *Br. Med. J.*, 1950, **2**, 1419; *Br. J. Anaesth.*, 1960, **32**, 132; Boulton, T. B. Paediatric anaesthesia and the Jackson Rees modification of Ayre's T-piece. 'Classical File', *Surv. Anesthesiol.*, 1985, **29**, 139
45. Snow, J. *Lond. Med. Gaz.*, 1850, **11**, 753; *ibid.*, **12**, 626
46. Kuhn, F. *Dtsch. Zeit. Chir.*, 1906, **81**, 63
47. Reinhold, H. In *Anaesthesia, Essays on its History*, edited by J. Rupreht and M. J. Van Lieburg, Springer-Verlag, Berlin, 1985
48. Jackson, D. E. *J. Lab. Clin. Med.*, 1915, **1**, 1 (reprinted in 'Classical File', *Surv. Anesthesiol.*, 1965, **98**, 9)
49. Waters, R. M. *Curr. Res. Anesth. Analg.*, 1924, **3**, 20
50. Waters, R. M. *Curr. Res. Anesth. Analg.*, 1926, **5**, 160; *Ann. Surg.*, 1936, **38**, 103; *Proc. Roy. Soc. Med.*, 1936, **30**, 11
51. Sword, B. C. *Curr. Res. Anesth. Analg.*, 1930, **9**, 198 (reprinted in 'Classical File', *Surv. Anesthesiol.*, 1981, **25**, 65)
52. Primrose, W. B. *Br. Med. J.*, 1934, **1**, 478; *ibid.*, **2**, 339
53. Waters, R. M. *Anesthesiology*, 1943, **4**, 596; Patterson, R. W. In *Anaesthesia, Essays on its History*, edited by J. Rupreht and M. J. Van Lieburg, Springer-Verlag, Berlin, 1985, pp.74, 167
54. Hewer, C. Langton, *Br. J. Anaesth.*, 1923–24, **1**, 113
55. See also Bendixen, H. H. *Acta Anaesthesiol. Scand.*, 1982, **26**, 279; Mushin, W. W., Rendell-Baker, L., Thompson, P. W. and Mapleson, W. W. *Automatic Ventilation of the Lungs*, 3rd edn, Blackwell, Oxford, 1980
56. Meltzer, S. J. *Med. Rec.*, 1917, **92**, 1
57. Northrup, W. P. *Med. Surg. Rep. Presbyterian Hosp., N. Y.*, 1896, **1**, 127
58. Matas, R. *Am. Med.*, 1902, **3**, 97
59. Sauerbruch, F. *Zbl. Chir.*, 1904, **31**, 146
60. Woollam, C. H. M. *Anaesthesia*, 1976, **31**, 537, 666
61. Thunberg, T. *Hyg. Rev. Uppsala*, 1924, **13**, 142; *Skand. Arch. Physiol.*, 1926, **48**, 80
62. Shaw, L. A. and Drinker, P. *J. Clin. Invest.*, 1929, **8**, 33; Drinker, P. and McKhann, C. F. *J. A. M. A.*, 1929, **92**, 1658
63. Frenckner, P. *Acta Otolaryngol. Scand.*, 1934, Suppl. 20, 3; Anderson, E., Crafoord, C. and Freckner, P. *Acta Otolaryngol.*, 1940, **28**, 95
64. Trier Mørch, E. *Proc. Roy. Soc. Med.*, 1947, **40**, 603
65. Pinson, K. B. and Bryce, A. G. *Br. J. Anaesth.*, 1944, **19**, 53
66. Musgrove, A. H. *Anaesthesia*, 1952, **7**, 77
67. Engström, C. G. *Br. Med. J.*, 1954, **2**, 666

6
Premedication

Before the introduction of anaesthesia

In the days before anaesthesia, both wine and opium were given to mitigate the terrors of surgery. Fallopius had given them a fairly bad reputation: 'If soporifics are weak, they will not help, if they are strong, they are exceedingly dangerous.' Wedel took a rather more lenient view: 'Opium in a moderate draught, given to the patient on the night preceding operation, for thus he bears the burning and cutting of the limb with a readier spirit, and various symptoms will be averted.'[1] The following description of an operation of those times serves to emphasize the vast change which anaesthesia brought:[2]

With a meek imploring look, and the startled air of a fawn, as her modest gaze meets the bold eyes fixed upon her, she is brought into the amphitheatre crowded with men anxious to see the shedding of her blood, and laid upon the table. With a knowledge and merciful regard of the agony which she is to suffer, opiates and stimulants have been freely given to her, which perhaps, at this stage, are again repeated. She is cheered by kind words and the information that it will soon be over, and she freed forever from what now afflicts her. She is enjoined to be calm and to keep quiet and still and, with assistance at hand to hold her struggling form, the operation is commenced.

But of what avail are all her attempts at fortitude? At the first clear crisp cut of the scalpel, agonising screams burst from her and with convulsive struggles she endeavours to leap from the table. But the force is nigh. Strong men throw themselves upon her and pinion her limbs. Shrieks upon shrieks make their horrible way into the stillness of the room, until the heart of the boldest sinks in his bosom like a lump of lead.

At length it is finished and, prostrated with pain, weak from her exertions, and bruised by the violence used, she is borne from the amphitheatre to her bed in the wards, to recover from the shock by slow degrees.

Richerand describes the use of opium as a preoperative medication (or even an intoxicant) for dislocations: 'Opium administered with a view to provoking sleep, or at least a state approaching intoxication, induces such an enfeeblement in the strength of the muscles that they cease to oppose reduction. One knows how easy it is to operate upon intoxicated persons.'[3] The use of opioids continued through into the early days of anaesthesia. Morton had used huge doses of opioids in a partially successful attempt to relieve the pain of dental extraction even before he introduced ether.[2] John Snow refers to laudanum given to a patient with tetanus in March 1858. Snow even attempted the use of opium as an antiemetic![4]

The use of opiates

Morphine had been introduced under the skin, using a vaccination lancet, by G. V. Lafargue of St. Emilion in 1836.[5] Claude Bernard recommended preoperative subcutaneous morphine in dogs to enhance the effect of chloroform with conspicuous success.[6] Nussbaum did the same with morphine intraoperatively during a tumour removal in 1864.[7] Labbé and Guyon reported excellent results of premedication with 20 mg morphine 'into the inner side of the thigh' in 1872.[8] Experiments with chloral premedication (thought to produce chloroform in the body) were made[9] and Oré gave it intravenously[10] but it was abandoned due to fatalities.

The word 'premedication' first appeared in print in an article by the American editor and anaesthetist Francis Hoeffer McMechan (1879–1939) in 1920.[11] Although drugs had been given by injection (the term 'hypodermic' was first used in 1859),[12] the technique of premedication was employed only infrequently during the 50 years following the introduction of anaesthesia. It was recommended by Bellamy Gardner[13] and Dudley Buxton (1855–1931) of University College Hospital in the UK,[14] and rules determining whether or not 'preliminary medication' should be used were published in 1911 in the USA.[15] In 1914 it was stated that preliminary medication was employed in 59% of hospitals in the USA.[16]

Papaveretum was prepared in 1909 by Hermann Sahli (1856–1933) of Berne and was marketed in Germany as Pantopon. Later, as Omnopon it became popular in the UK.[17] Pethidine, synthesized in 1939 by Schaumann and Eisleb in Germany during a search for a substitute for atropine,[18] was first used in premedication by Schlungbaum[19] and in the USA in 1943.[20]

Anticholinergic drugs

Atropine

Atropine (from Atropos, the oldest of the Three Fates who severed the threads of life, which were spun by Clotho and mixed, those of good and evil fortune, by Lachesis) is the alkaloid of the *Atropa belladonna* or deadly nightshade. In the mid-nineteenth century it was used as a mydriatic, to relieve asthma or colic and for epilepsy. It had been combined with morphine in 1858[21] in the belief that they antagonized each other's side-effects, and was first suggested in 1880 by E. A. Sharpey-Schaffer (1850–1935), Edinburgh physiologist, for the specific effect of reducing vagal tone during chloroform anaesthesia. It was also advocated by Dudley Buxton (1855–1935), London anaesthetist, 35 years later to inhibit secretions during ether anaesthesia.[22] It was not used in premedication before 1890, although it was given, as the extract, per rectum, in Vienna, in 1861 to control patients resistant to chloroform.[23] The patient reported was unrousable for 12 hours, possibly the first case of central anticholinergic syndrome. More latterly it has usually been prepared from the plant *Duboisia myoporoides*. Atropine was first synthesized by Richard Willstaetter (1872–1942) in 1896, and again by Robert Robinson in 1917.

Hyoscine

Hyoscine was in favour as a sedative (without constipating properties) long before anaesthesia and is referred to by Snow[24] as tincture hyoscyamus. He does not appear to have used its significant antiemetic properties, in spite of frequent mention of operative and postoperative vomiting! The name 'scopolamine' was derived from *Scopolia carniolica*, the plant from which it was first isolated. The plant itself was named after Johannes Antonius Scopoli (1723–88), a physician from Carniola, a province in Slovenia.[25] It was also derived (especially in nineteenth century English use) from *Hyoscyamus niger* (henbane). Morphine and hyoscine were combined in 1868,[26] producing excellent sedation, analgesia and antiemesis. This was a characteristic triumph of pharmacological knowledge applied to clinical practice.

Hyoscine was isolated in 1873.[27] It was originally used as a mixture of laevo– and dextro-rotatory alkaloids, and achieved a reputation for unreliability. When it was discovered that only the laevo form was pharmacologically active, this was prepared and sold in Germany under the name of scopolamine, where it soon became widely used. A pioneer of its use in the UK was Dudley Wilmot Buxton. In the very early 1900s it became popular for preoperative medication because it dried secretions, was sedative, antiemetic and amnesic – a superb combination. It was used, together with morphine, before anaesthesia in 1900 by Schneiderlinn.[28] It was also used around this time to produce amnesia in labour (twilight sleep).[29]

Glycopyrronium

Over half a century was to elapse before the next advance in drying and vagolytic agents – glycopyrronium. This was synthesized by Franko and Lunsford,[30] and first used in anaesthesia by Boawright, Newell and colleagues in 1970.[31] Its advantage was that, as a quaternary ammonium compound, it did not cross the blood–brain barrier, and so did not cause central anticholinergic syndrome, an occasional problem with atropine and hyoscine.

The use of any anticholinergic premedication has become much less important with the advent of the fluorocarbon volatile agents which cause less problems with bronchial secretions.[32] Indeed in many clinical situations the various disadvantages of atropine (need for an injection, interference with sweating, dry mouth, tachycardia, ileus, and perhaps more viscous secretions) can outweigh its supposed advantages, and all such anticholinergic drugs are used less commonly today.

Other premedicants

Barbiturates were used as premedicants as soon as they were available. Boyd reported the use of Nembutal in over 1000 patients in 1932.[33] The benzodiazepines also rapidly became popular for premedication in the 1970s in Western countries. They had the advantage that they were reliable when given orally, produced amnesia as well as sedation, relaxed muscle and were not subject to the restrictions that make the administration of controlled drugs more difficult. An early one, lorazepam[34] was long-acting, and all the patients for an operating list could be premedicated at the same time – about an hour before the list commenced! The development of benzodiazepines is described in Chapter 7.

For a further discussion of the evolvement of premedication, see Shearer, W. *Br. J. Anaesth.*, 1960, **32**; 554 *ibid.*, 1961, **33**, 219

References

1. Wedel, G. W. *Opiologica ad mentem academiae naturae curiosorum*, 1682, Jena, pp.129–130
2. Rice, N. *Trials of a Public Benefactor*, New York, 1859
3. Richerand, A. *Nosographie Chirurgicale*, Paris, 1812, **3**, 181
4. Ellis, R. H. (ed.) Facsimile edition of Snow, J. *On Narcotism by the Inhalation of Vapours*, Royal Society of Medicine, London, 1991, p.56
5. Lafargue, G. V. C. R.. *Acad. Sci. Paris*, 1836, **2**, 397; *Bull. Acad. Med. Paris*, 1836, **1**, 13
6. Bernard, C. *Dent. Rev.*, 1864, **NS1**, 203
7. Nussbaum, J. N. von. *Med. Times Lond.*, 1864, **1**, 259

8. Labbé, A. and Guyon, P. *C. R.. Acad. Sci. Paris*, 1872, **74**, 627

9. Annotation, *C. R.. Acad. Sci. Paris*, 1869, **69**, 486, 979

10. Oré, J.C. *C. R.. Acad. Sci. Paris*, 1874, **78**, 515, 651

11. McMechan, F. H. *Am. J. Surg.*, 1920, suppl. 34, 123; *Lancet*, 1928, **2**, 1252

12. Hunter, C. *Br. Med. J.*, 1859, **i**, 19

13. Bellamy Gardner, H. *Br. Med. J.*, 1910, **2**, 766

14. Buxton, W. D. *Proc. R. Soc. Med.*, 1908–09, **2**, 60; *ibid.*, 1911, **4**, 53

15. Collins, C. U. *J.A.M.A.*, 1911, **56**, 47

16. Gwathmey, J. T. *Anesthesia*, D. Appleton & Co, New York and London, 1914, p.847

17. Leipoldt, C. L. *Lancet*, 1911, **1**, 368; Kerri Szanto, M. *Can. Anaesth. Soc. J.*, 1974, **23**, 239

18. Schaumann, O. and Eisleb, O. *Dtsch. Med. Wochenschr.*, 1939, **65**, 967

19. Schlungbaum, H. *Med. Klin.*, 1939, **35**, 1259

20. Rovenstine, E. A. and Battermann, R. I. *Anesthesiology*, 1943, **4**, 126

21. Bell, B. *Edinb. Med. J.*, 1858–59, **NS4**, 1

22. Kessel, J. *Anaesth. Intensive Care*, 1974, **2**, 77

23. Pitha, J. *Medical Times, Lond.*, 1861, **2**, 121

24. Ellis, R. H. (ed.) *The Casebooks of Dr John Snow*, Wellcome Institute for the History of Medicine, London, 1995

25. Soban, D. *Progress in Anaesthesiology*, Excerpta Medica Foundation, Amsterdam, 1970, p.193

26. Harley, J. *Br. Med. J.*, 1868, **1**, 319, 343

27. Ladenburg, A. *Ann. Chem. Pharmac.*, 1881, **206**, 274

28. Schneiderlinn, J. *Aertz. Mitt. a. Baden*, 1900, **54**, 104

29. Gauss, C. J. *Arch. Gynaek.*, 1906, **78**, 579

30. Franko, B. V. and Lunsford, C. D. *J. Med. Pharm. Chem.*, 1960, **11**, 523

31. Boawright, C. F., Newell, R. C. *et al. Am. Acad. Ophthal. Otolaryngol.*, 1970, **74**, 1139

32. Holt, A. T. *Lancet*, 1962, **2**, 984

33. Boyd, A. M. *St. Bart's Hosp. Rep.*, 1932, **65**, 283

34. Norris, W. and Wallace, P. G. M. *Br. J. Anaesth.*, 1971, **43**, 785

7

Intravenous drugs in anaesthesia

Intravenous anaesthetic agents

A few far-sighted pioneers conceived the principle of this approach in the seventeenth century, but lacked the technology and the availability of suitable agents. The time delay between the pioneers and the advent of the appropriate technology was two centuries! After this it was a further five or six decades before the drugs were created to make intravenous anaesthesia popular. The arrival of hexobarbitone in 1931 marked the birth of a new age of anaesthesia in which intravenous induction and supplementation became the norm, resulting in more comfort for the patient, but not necessarily more safety (see below).

Johann Sigismund Elsholtz (1623–88), a German physician, injected opium intravenously to produce unconsciousness in 1665[108]. Francis Rynd (1801–61) of Dublin in 1845[1] used a trocar and cannula with morphine for the treatment of trigeminal neuralgia, but he did not use a syringe. Pierre-Cyprien Oré (1828–91),[2] Professor of Physiology at Bordeaux, used chloral hydrate intravenously in 1872 in a patient suffering from tetanus, and even used it to allow minor surgery. It proved too dangerous. Alexander Wood (1817–84)[3] of Edinburgh was the true founder of hypodermic anaesthetic medication. He used a Ferguson syringe (syringe from Greek *syrinx* = a tube or pipe). The hypodermic syringe and needle were not, as often supposed, invented by the Frenchman, Charles Gabriel Pravaz (1791–1853) of Lyons.[4] He used a syringe whose piston was advanced on a spiral thread to allow the steady injection of iron perchloride into an aneurysmal artery. The Record syringe of metal and glass was introduced about 1906 in Berlin, and the French Luer followed it.[5] The first indwelling intravenous needles to remain patent for multiple injections were described by Olovson and Torsten Gordh in the 1940s.[6]

Intravenous ether had been used in animals by Nikolai Ivanovitch Pirogoff (1810–81) in Russia in 1847, a year after Morton's use of ether by inhalation. It was used in surgery in 1909 by Ludwig

Burkhardt (1872–1922), Nuremburg surgeon, with some successes but many failures. A 2.5–5% solution in normal saline or in 5% glucose was used. He also used chloroform in this way. Intravenous hedonal was used in 1905 by Krawkow of St. Petersburg, Russia[7] and in 1912 by Max Page in London.

Barbituric acid was synthesized by Adolf v. Baeyer (1835–1917) of Munich in 1864 but its narcotic effects were not realized at that time. Later, also in Munich, a barbiturate was synthesized by Emil Fischer (1852–1918) and Joseph Friederich von Mering (1849–1908) in 1903.[8] This was diethyl barbituric acid or Veronal. Phenobarbitone was discovered in 1912. Somnifaine was the first barbiturate to be given intravenously. It was a combination of diethyl and diallyl barbituric acids, and was used in France by Bardet in 1924.[9]

Noel and Souttar used intravenous paraldehyde in 1913.[10] Intravenous morphine and hyoscine were employed for 'twilight sleep' in 1916.[11] In 1927 Bumm introduced Pernocton,[12] while Zerfas, in the USA, used sodium amytal intravenously[13] 2 years later. This was soon followed by pentobarbitone or Nembutal.[14] Magill was the first to demonstrate this clinically in Britain.[15] John Silas Lundy[16] (1890–1974), of the Mayo Clinic, attempted to popularize Nembutal in the USA in 1931. Martin Kirschner (1879–1942) of Heidelberg gave Avertin (bromethol) intravenously in 1929[17] with moderate success. Great credit belongs to these pioneer experimenters for foresight and courage in seeking to extend the frontiers of anaesthesia. They did not achieve their aim but they laid important foundations of pharmacological understanding for a later generation. None of these early beginnings was really successful, and the world of anaesthesia awaited the discovery of better drugs.

Hexobarbitone (Figure 7.1) was the breakthrough. It was the first drug to make intravenous anaesthesia popular and was used in 1932 by Helmut Weese (1897–1954) (Figure 7.2), Professor of Pharmacology at Dusseldorf and Director of Pharmacology at Bayer (Wuppertal-Elberfeld). The historical significance of this lay in the happy partnership between academia and big business, a model which has been copied many times since, to the benefit of humankind. He was the true father of intravenous anaesthesia. Hexobarbitone was synthesized in 1931 by Kropp and Taub in Elberfeld. Weese reported its use together with Walter Scharpff the next year.[18] It was first given in Great Britain in 1933 by Ronald Jarman (1898–1973) and L. Abel in London.[19]

Thiopentone (pentothal sodium) was synthesized in 1932 by Ernest Henry Volwiler and Donalee Tabern[20] and introduced into clinical practice by Waters of Madison on 3 March 1934,[21] and by John Silas Lundy (1894–1973) (Figure 7.3) of the Mayo Clinic on 18 June 1934.[22] Lundy was the more influential, probably because of his

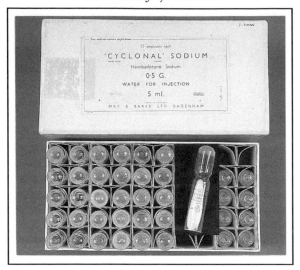

Figure 7.1   Hexobarbitone ampoules

earlier experience with the less successful nembutal. It was first used in Great Britain by Jarman and Abel in 1935.[23] Its fate in the body and distribution were described by Brodie in 1950.[24] Thiopentone was originally employed as the sole anaesthetic and if used by the inexperienced under adverse conditions can cause circulatory collapse, e.g. at Pearl Harbor on 9 December 1941, although this particular episode has been re-evaluated.[25] Intermittent dosage, along with nitrous oxide and oxygen, was first described by Geoffrey Stephen William Organe (1908–85) and Broad in 1938.[26]

Methohexitone, a methyl barbiturate, was first described by S. M. Chernish *et al.* in 1956,[29] and first used by Stoelting in the USA in 1957.[30] It was introduced into Britain by Dundee and Moore in 1961.[31] It is still in relatively common use.

Many intravenous anaesthetic agents were tried in the postwar years but did not survive. Examples included **hydroxydione** in 1955; **propanidid** in 1966; **gamma-hydroxybutyric acid** in 1960 and **alphaxalone/alphadolone (Althesin)** in 1971.[32] This was part of the natural evolution of intravenous anaesthesia and this series of drugs has eventually led to the excellent agents available at the end of the twentieth century. It is a tribute to the excellence of thiopentone that it has survived 60 years and remains in common use.

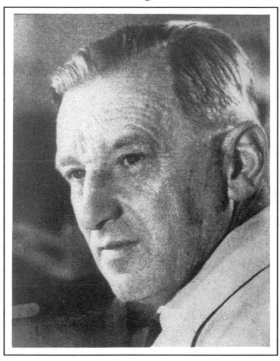

Figure 7.2   Helmut Weese (1897–1954)

Deserves an honoured place in the history of anaesthesia as the first man to make intravenous induction a safe and practical procedure. Born in Munich into a family originating from the German part of Poland, and the son of a lecturer in the history of art. When he was nine, the family moved to Berne where his father became a privatdozent at the University. Switzerland had a great influence on his development. Decided to study medicine and attended the Universities of Berne, Zurich and Munich where he qualified. His first post was in internal medicine under von Romberg, and then he changed to pharmacology in 1925 and worked with W. Straub. Did well in the new discipline and in his own turn became privatdozent. Paid particular attention to the study of digitalis, wrote a book on it and, as a result, became well known both inside and outside Germany to physicians as well as to pharmacologists. When in 1928, F. Eicholtz who had previously described the effects of bromethol (Avertin) moved to Konigsberg and then to Heidelberg, Weese followed him as Director of Pharmacology at the Farbwerk Bayer at Wuppertal-Elberfeld, and as lecturer at the University of Cologne. Appointed professor there in 1936. Not a purely academic scientist, he always strove to direct his energies to the relief of his fellow men. In 1931, Kropp and Taub synthesized a new barbiturate, hexobarbitone, later to become known as Evipan. Weese saw that this might be the long-awaited short-acting and safe agent for induction of anaesthesia, and at once set about investigating it both in the laboratory and personally in the operating theatre. Soon able to show that it fulfilled his expectations and in 1932 he published his results, thus becoming the undisputed creator of practical clinical modern intravenous anaesthesia. Won recognition at the International Congress of Anesthesia at New York in 1938, during which he was elected as an honorary member.

During World War II, Weese, who was Consultant Pharmacologist to the Armed Forces, investigated the possibility of producing a synthetic plasma volume expander, and as a result, polyvinyl pyrrolidone (Periston, polyvidone) became available and saved many lives. Also devoted time to investigating the application of phenothiazines to clinical anaesthesia, following the stimulus of the Frenchmen, Laborit and Huguenard. With Hans Killian he wrote a book on anaesthesia, *Die Narkose*. Practised both anaesthesia and pharmacology and was honoured by members of both specialities. Used his considerable influence to advance the status of anaesthesia in postwar Germany. Died following a fall from a chair in his laboratory, an unusual event in a man well used to climbing in the high Alps. (For his obituary, see Killian, H. *Der Anaesthesist*, 1954, Band 3; Heft 2. 97. Translation, Dr Heinrich Niehoff.)

Etomidate was synthesized and studied by Janssen and co-workers in 1971 and used in man by Alfred Doenicke of Munich and colleagues in 1973. It had one great advantage over barbiturates – it did not depress the circulation. It continues in use as an induction agent mainly because of this feature. It was found to depress adrenal function when used as a continuous infusion in the intensive care unit, in the Western Infirmary, Glasgow, in 1983.[33]

A significant step forward was the introduction of **propofol**, whose first reported use was in 1977.[34] The original product was dissolved in Cremophor EL,[35] but this was changed to soybean oil emulsion because of the side-effects of cremophor. The history of intravenous anaesthesia might have been very different if other manufacturers had taken this simple step. This drug has now risen to a prominent position as an anaesthetic induction agent. It was also a powerful trigger for the development of total intravenous anaesthesia in the 1980s. It is relatively safe, has a quick offset, and some antiemetic properties. One other great advantage is the suppression of laryngeal reflexes by this drug.

Other drugs used for intravenous anaesthesia

Promethazine, a drug thought to stabilize cell membranes when synthesized, was first used in anaesthesia in the 'lytic cocktail' (a form of very deep sedation). In the mid–1950s work on the existing tranquillizers was extended. These included chlorpromazine, reserpine and meprobamate.

Benzodiazepines had been studied in Cracow, Poland in the 1930s[36] and elsewhere. Chlordiazepoxide was prepared in 1960 and named Librium, the pharmacology having been worked out by Randall. It was first used clinically in 1961. The first reported use of benzodiazepine as an intravenous anaesthetic in the UK was in 1966 (diazepam). The group also included temazepam (Normison) and lorazepam (Ativan) which became popular oral premedicants

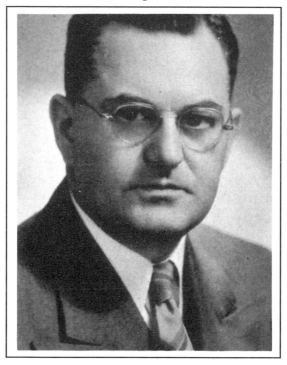

Figure 7.3   John Silas Lundy (1894–1973)[27]

Dr Lundy of the Mayo Clinic, Rochester, Minnesota, had a great influence on the speciality of anaesthesia, particularly as the pioneer of the use of thiopentone. Born in Seattle, Washington, the son of a doctor. Took an arts degree in 1917 and qualified in medicine from the Rush Medical College in Chicago 2 years later. After serving as a resident in Chicago hospitals, returned to his birthplace and entered general practice. In April 1924 he was invited to become head of the Department of Anesthesiology at the Mayo Clinic and this he directed for the next 28 years, although his connection with the clinic did not end until 1959. Became professor in the Mayo Graduate School of Medicine in 1934 and was one of the founders of the American Board of Anesthesiology. Was a prolific writer, and this, together with the worldwide reputation of the Mayo Clinic where he worked, soon carried his name throughout the USA and Europe. Established the first laboratory of gross anatomy to be used at the clinic, and this was important for his teaching of the techniques of regional analgesia which had been stimulated there by Gaston Labat. In 1925 he developed the theory and practice of 'balanced anesthesia'[28] and although Waters of Madison used thiopentone $3\frac{1}{2}$ months before he did (Lundy used it on 18 June 1934), Lundy continued throughout his professional life to advocate its use. It is largely due to his efforts that intravenous induction spread so widely. In 1942 he opened the first post-anaesthesia observation room (recovery room) at St. Mary's Hospital, Rochester. In 1935 he established the first blood bank in the USA at Rochester. Was the author of the textbook *Clinical Anesthesia*, published in 1942, one of the first authoritative volumes dealing with the so-called 'modern anaesthesia'. Received many medals, awards and honours from academic bodies throughout the world. Retired first to Chicago and later to Seattle where he continued to practise anaesthesia.

in the 1970s, and midazolam (Hypnovel). They remain in wide-spread use as sedatives, tranquillizers and amnesics, but anaesthesia awaits the appearance of a much shorter-acting agent of this class.

Neurolept analgesia was introduced in 1959, when the term 'neurolepsis' was coined by Delay,[37] and 'neurolept analgesia' was developed by J. A. De Castro and Mundeleer of Brussels in the same year.[38] A development of the concepts of artificial hibernation, neurovegetative block and ataralgesia, the neuroleptic agents used in anaesthesia were chemically based on methyl ethylamine and were related to gamma-hydroxybutyric acid (GABA). The addition of potent short-acting analgesics changed what was otherwise a rather clumsy technique into a much more reliable one, and which had great potential for use in surgical manoeuvres. **Fentanyl** and **alfentanil**, first used in 1981, were the agents of choice for this, having been developed by Janssen for swiftness of onset and durations well matched to a wide range of surgical procedures.

A parallel development was the introduction of the powerful analgesic, **ketamine**. A related compound, phencyclidine (Sernyl; 'angel dust') had been synthesized by Victor Maddox of Detroit, investigated by Chen of Ann Arbor[39] and was used in anaesthesia, but had to be withdrawn because of the high incidence of hallucinations. Ketamine was synthesized by Stevens of Detroit and tested on volunteers from a state prison in Michigan in 1964. It was used in anaesthesia in 1965 by Domino and Corssen.[40] Ketamine has been used for intradural analgesia in war surgery,[41] and can also be given orally. It, too has stood the test of time, and is used throughout the world as a powerful analgesic, sedative and bronchodilator, which retains circulatory stability in the elderly and frail patient.[42]

Pregnenolone, an agent with high therapeutic ratio and cardiovascular stability, was investigated in 1992.[43] Its position in the therapeutic armamentarium remains to be confirmed.

With the above powerful and safe intravenous anaesthetics, there were situations when they might be preferred to gaseous or volatile agents. **Total intravenous anaesthesia** gained popularity in the 1980s with the advent of propofol, and automated infusion programs were written to control their administration.[44] Crude clockwork syringe pumps were in use in the 1960s for infusion of hypotensive drugs and were developed into sophisticated syringe drivers in the 1980s. They also found wide application in intensive care and other areas of clinical practice (Figure 7.4). The advent of propofol, and the use of infusions in many areas of medicine, was a powerful stimulus for the development of the electronic pumps that began in the 1980s.

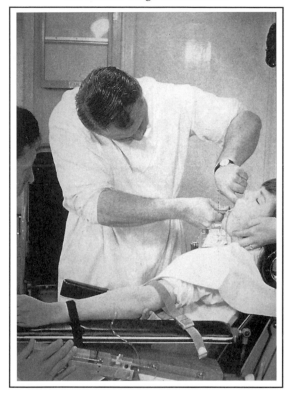

Figure 7.4 Total intravenous outpatient dental anaesthesia in the 1960s

Sedation techniques or 'sedoanalgesia'

These combinations of local analgesia and light sedation (often aided by some forms of sensory deprivation, e.g. earmuffs, eyeshades, etc.) had their origins in the early days of anaesthesia, especially in obstetric analgesia, and are frequently referred to by Snow.[45] The analgesia was produced by very light planes of general anaesthesia before the introduction of cocaine.

The benzodiazepines opened a new chapter in the management of sedation for investigative procedures in the 1960s because of the quality of sedation and amnesia. Ketamine added the possibility of profound analgesia. Because of the side-effects of these drugs, and the need to monitor and control the patient's physiology during such procedures, these techniques often needed much care from a second doctor in attendance. The use of opiates by an 'operator-sedator' was proscribed by the 'Guidelines on sedation by non-anaesthetists', of the Royal College of Surgeons of England in 1993.

Muscle relaxants

Background

The first hint of these drugs to the ears of the Western world was in **1596** when Sir Walter Raleigh (1552–1618) mentioned an 'arrow poison' in his book *Discovery of the Large, Rich, and Beautiful Empire of Guiana*. It is possible that the poison he described was not curare at all.[46]

Over 200 years later, in **1812**, Sir Benjamin Collins Brody (1783–1862)[47] experimented with curare.[48] He was the first to show that artificial respiration could maintain life in curarized animals. The source of curare was from bark, leaves and vines of *Chondroden-dron tomentosum* growing near the upper reaches of the Amazon and had long been used by Amazonian Indians to poison the heads of their arrows. They transported it in bamboo tubes, hence the name tubocurarine. Curare had been brought to Europe by Charles Waterton (1782–1865) in 1812. He was squire of Walton Hall, Yorkshire, and wrote *Wanderings in South America* in 1825. He described a classic experiment in which he kept a curarized she-ass alive by artificial ventilation with a bellows through a tracheostomy.[49]

In **1850** the great French physiologist Claude Bernard (1813–78),[50] stimulated by François Magendie (1783–1855), laid the scientific foundation for use of relaxants by showing that curare acts by paralysing the myoneural junction. This led to his discovery of the concept of the motor end-plate. George Harley (1829–96) (of ACE anaesthetic mixture fame) showed that curare (wourali) was an efficient antidote to strychnine poisoning and also a treatment for the spasms of tetanus.[51]

Therapeutic use of relaxants

A decade after the anaesthetic use of ether, in **1858**, Lewis Albert Sayer (1820–1900) used curare to treat tetanus in New York,[52] and in **1862** curare was used by Chisholm, in the American Civil War. Thus this relaxant was used in disease long before it was used for anaesthesia. Another foundation was laid for muscle relaxants in anaesthesia in **1864**, when physostigmine was isolated from the calabar bean by Sir T. R. Fraser (1841–1920), a Scottish pharmacologist who also showed that atropine counteracts its muscarinic effects.[53]

By **1872**, curare was in use by Demme for the treatment of tetanus, and in **1894** R. Boehm (1844–1926), a German pharmacologist, separated curare into 'pot', 'gourd' and 'tube' curare according to the method used for storing it by the South American Indians. In 1897 he isolated highly active extracts from calabash curare.[54] The discovery of the anticurare action of physostigmine in **1900** by Jacob Pal (1863–1936)[55] completed the basic foundations on which relaxants would be used later in the century.

Physostigmine was used in animal experimentation in 1909,[56] and in **1912** curare first entered the anaesthetic arena and was used by Arthur Läwen (1876–1958)* of Konigsberg[57] in an effort to reduce the amount of ether employed in abdominal surgery with intermittent positive pressure ventilation. The purpose of this was to reduce the incidence of postoperative pulmonary complications which were thought to be due to the ether vapour. The doses of curare used were subparalytic, producing relaxation of the abdominal wall but not preventing respiratory movement of the diaphragm.

Why were anaesthetists tragically slow to realize the benefits of muscle relaxants? It was a century after Brody's classic experiment, and over half a century after the first gaseous anaesthetic, before curare was first used in anaesthesia. The spirit of experimentation and innovation in other matters was strong among anaesthetists of this period, and they were not noted for any innate conservatism. More probably they were horrified by the prospect of producing apnoea.

Some of the physiological actions of acetylcholine were described in **1914** by Sir Henry Dale (1875–1968)[59] and were the essential stimulus to further work. The development of relaxants and antidotes was gathering pace, and in **1931** neostigmine methylsulphate (Prostigmine) was synthesized by Aeschlimann and Reinert.[60] They

---

* **Arthur Läwen (1876–1958)**

Born in Waldheim in Saxony and qualified at Leipzig in 1900. Became a pupil of Heinrich Braun (1862–1935) in Leipzig and later of Friedrich Trendelenburg (1844–1924) and Erwin Payr (1871–1976) of Griefswald. Held senior posts at Leipzig and Marburg and was appointed Professor of Surgery at Königsberg in East Prussia where his chief work was done, including his pioneering introduction of curare into clinical anaesthesia. This work was interrupted by World War I. Was also the first to describe paravertebral conduction anaesthesia, and in 1910 he was the first to show that extradural analgesia was a safe and practical form of pain relief in pelvic and abdominal surgery. For this he used large volumes of 1.5% or 2% procaine solution with sodium bicarbonate, injected through the sacral hiatus.[58] Did a great deal to popularize local analgesia, tracheal intubation and artificial respiration. After 1945 he became a refugee from East Germany, having lost his sons, his possessions and his university chair during the war. Died in 1958, aged 82.

showed that it had an anticurare action twice as powerful as physostigmine.

The first therapeutic use of curare in the UK (the treatment of tetanus), was at Cambridge in **1934** by Cole,[61] and later that year Dale demonstrated that acetylcholine was responsible for neuromuscular transmission, an effect blocked by curare.[62] In **1935** King (1887–1956)[63], of London, working in Sir Henry Dale's laboratory, isolated *d*-tubocurarine chloride from the crude drug and established its chemical structure. Ranyard West used this in the treatment of tetanus.[64] Dale further showed that a motor nerve liberates acetylcholine from the dense projections in the nerve terminal at the myoneural junction on the arrival of a nerve impulse,[65] in **1936**. Two years after this, Richard C. Gill (1902–58), an American explorer, obtained supplies of crude curare and later drew attention to the drug in his book *White Water and Blue Magic*, New York, 1940.

Abram Elting Bennett,[66] of Omaha (Nebraska) then employed curare in **1939** to modify metrazol-induced convulsive therapy. (It was later used by Harold Palmer,[67] of Hill End Hospital, St. Albans, Hertfordshire, to modify ECT.) Bennett arranged for crude curare to be given by Gill to McIntyre of the University of Nebraska who first standardized the drug.

Widespread use of relaxants in anaesthesia

The interest of a drug company prompted the clinical breakthrough for which the world of anaesthesia was waiting. Harold Randall Griffith (1894–1985),* assisted by his resident Enid Johnson (later of

---

* **Harold Randall Griffith (1894–1985)**[68]

Born near Montreal on 25 July 1894 and obtained the BA (Magill) in 1914 and the MD CM in 1922. In this year he also married. The following year he obtained the MD in homeopathic medicine from the Hahnemann Medical College in Philadelphia. Before graduating in medicine he served with distinction as a stretcher-bearer in the Canadian Army and was awarded the Military Medal for bravery in World War I. An interest in anaesthesia developed early in his career and after a time he became chief anaesthetist at the Montreal Homeopathic Hospital where his father had been Medical Director and his brother had been Surgeon-in-Chief. Spent his active professional life here until his retirement in 1966. Before the days of relaxants he developed an expertise in tracheal intubation and, along with Dr Ralph Waters of Madison, became a world expert on the use of the then new agent cyclopropane. As anaesthesia advanced, he became involved in its academic side and was appointed Professor of Anaesthesia and Chairman of the Department at Magill University. Held high office in the International Anesthesia Research Society and was a founder member of the World Federation of Societies of Anesthesiology and President of its First Congress held in Holland in 1955, and at its Second Congress held in Toronto in 1959 he was elected permanent Founder-President.

Harold Griffith was a much loved man of modest disposition who was known to his younger colleagues as Uncle Harold. In later life he received many honours and distinctions including the Hickman Medal from the Royal Society of Medicine in London in 1956, and he was the only non-US citizen to receive the Distinguished Service Award from the American Society of Anesthesiology. Harold Griffith died aged 90 of Parkinson's disease on 7 May 1985.

Nova Scotia), used curare intravenously in **1942** (the commercial preparation Intocostrin, prepared by Horace Holaday) at the suggestion of Dr Lewis Wright of E. M. Squibb Co.,[69] deliberately to give relaxation during surgery, on 23 January in Montreal, Canada. The patient, a man weighing 150 lb (68 kg), underwent an interval appendicectomy under cyclopropane anaesthesia at the Homeopathic Hospital (later the Queen Elizabeth Hospital) in Montreal. This was a famous day in the history of anaesthesia,[70] not because something new was done, but because the anaesthetists of the world finally appreciated the advantages of muscle relaxants as part of the anaesthetic sequence.

The history of muscle relaxants has, from this point onwards, been to the great credit of many drug companies. Development passed increasingly from practising doctors to the research laboratories of the pharmaceutical industry. Messrs Squibb obtained their supply of curare from R. C. Gill who brought it back from his expedition to Ecuador. The extraction of tubocurarine from *Chondrodendron tomentosum* in **1943** by Wintersteiner,[71] provided the source of the drug for clinical use.

The same year saw the first publication of Stuart Chester Cullen (1909–79), a US pioneer of its use.[72] When given a sample of the preparation 'Intocostrin', Cullen first tried it on animals, and producing apnoea, was not able easily to ventilate them artificially, and so did not proceed to use it on humans. Griffith was also given a sample, but as he was familiar with the management of apnoea due to cyclopropane by using intermittent positive pressure ventilation, he did not find the apnoea caused by curare to be a problem. Thus he rightly claimed priority for the introduction of relaxants into anaesthetic practice.[73]

The earliest mention of the use of curare with unsupplemented nitrous oxide and oxygen was in **1944** by Waters in abdominal surgery[74] and also by Harroun in thoracic surgery.[75] The first reported use in Britain of curare (Intocostrin) in routine anaesthesia was in **1945** by Barnett Mallinson.[76] T. C. Gray (1913–) and John Halton (1904–69) of Liverpool were active in establishing the position of curare in Britain[77] from **1946**, but initially used only subparalytic doses without stopping spontaneous respiration.

The following year, Bovet described **gallamine triethiodide**.[78] This was used clinically in France by Huguenard and Boué in 1948[79] and by Mushin in 1949 in Britain.[80] At the same time, Neff published an influential article describing use of gas, oxygen, pethidine and curare.[81] The historical significance of this (and the subsequent Liverpool technique) was that they finally had the courage to abolish spontaneous respiration, making the patients entirely dependent on the hands of the anaesthetist. This went against traditional teaching on ether and chloroform anaesthesia.

In **1948 decamethonium** was described by Barlow and Ing[82] and by William Drummond Macdonald Paton (1917–) and Eleanor Zaimis (1915–82).[83] Other depolarizing relaxants, the *bis*-choline esters of succinic acid, were described by Daniel Bovet in **1949**[84] and by J. C. Castillo and Edwin de Beer[85] in **1950**. **Suxamethonium chloride** had been prepared and reported in the medical literature as early as **1906** by Reid Hunt (1870–1948) and R. Taveau of Boston.[86] As with curare, it took several decades for anaesthetists to adopt the use of this drug in clinical practice. Suxamethonium was first used in anaesthesia in **1951** by von Dardel, in Stockholm[87] and by Otto Mayerhofer in Vienna.[88] Cyril Fredrick Scurr then introduced it into Britain.[89]

A nerve stimulator was first used to assess neuromuscular transmission in man in 1949.[90] Electrical responses to nerve stimulation were recorded in 1952 on an Electro-Myo-Graph.[91] Mechanical responses to nerve stimulation were also recorded.[92] Prolonged apnoea after suxamethonium was found to be associated with an abnormal cholinesterase value by J. G. Bourne of London and his colleagues in 1952,[93] the hereditary nature of which was shown by Forbat[94] in 1953.

A sensational article by H. K. Beecher (1907–76) and D. P. Todd in 1954 suggested that the use of relaxants increased deaths due to anaesthesia nearly sixfold.[95] This was, of course, completely disproved. It has also to be remembered that the use of relaxants allowed surgery to be performed on very much sicker patients.

W. D. M. Paton made the distinction between depolarizing and non-depolarizing relaxants[96] in 1956. The curare-like action of aminoglycoside antibiotics (Neomycin) was first reported[97] in the same year.

In **1958** a new relaxant from *Strychnos toxifera*, later named **alcuronium**, was described[98] and first used in man[99] in **1961**. **Pancuronium** was synthesized in **1964** by Savage and Hewett, and used clinically,[100] following pharmacological investigations in 1966.[101] The correct structure of the tubocurarine molecule was finally worked out[102] in **1970**. By **1977** Michael Tunstall had developed the isolated forearm technique for detecting unplanned awareness during relaxant anaesthesia,[103] a technique which remains in use two decades later.

Vecuronium was introduced by Durant *et al.*[104] in **1979**. This was an historical event in that the molecule of pancuronium was deliberately altered to enable the liver to metabolize the drug more rapidly. It has proved a great success. **Atracurium** was used in man[105] the following year. These two relaxants have replaced most of those in former use, because they are shorter acting, more predictable and more easily reversed.

Mivacurium was introduced in **1993**, a 'designer' non-depolarizing relaxant with a duration of action of around 10 min,[106] which was metabolized by serum cholinesterase. Onset and recovery were even faster in children. In **1994 rocuronium** was introduced, another 'designer' non-depolarizing relaxant of rapid onset, approaching that of suxamethonium. Reduced receptor affinity enabled higher extracellular concentrations of drug, with consequent faster equilibration[107] with the biophase.

For further information on the history of relaxants, see Cullen, S. C. *Anesthesiology*, 1947, **8**, 479; Robbins, B. H. and Lundy, J. S. *Anesthesiology*, 1947, **8**, 252; McIntyre, A. R. *Curare; Its History, Nature and Clinical Use*, University of Chicago Press, Chicago, 1947; Thomas, K. B. *Curare. Its History and Usage*, Pitman, London, 1964; Stovner, J. In *Muscle Relaxants*, edited by Katz, L., Excerpta Medica, Amsterdam, 1975, Chap. 10; Crul, J. F. *Acta Anaesthesiol. Scand.*, 1982, **26**, 409; Humble, R. M. The Gill Merritt expedition. *Anesthesiology*, 1982, **57**, 519; Dorkin, H. R. Suxamethonium, the development of a modern drug from 1906 to the present day. *Med. Hist.*, 1982, **26**, 145.

References

1. Rynd, F. *Dublin Med. Press*, 1845, **13**, 167
2. Oré, P. C. *Bull. Soc. Chirurg.*, 1872, **1**, 400; see also Sabathié, M. and Delperier, A. *Progress in Anaesthesiology*, Excerpta Medica, Amsterdam, 1970, p.841
3. Wood, A. *Edin. Med. Surg. J.*, 1855, **82**, 265; Boulton, T. B. 'Classical File', *Surv. Anesthesiol.*, 1984, **28**, 346–354
4. Pravaz, C. G. *C. R. Séances Acad. Sci.*, 1853. **36**, 88
5. Howard-Jones, N. J. *J. Hist. Med.*, 1947, **2**, 201
6. Olovson, T. *Der Chirurg*, 1940, **12**; Gordh, T. *Anesthesiology*, 1945, **6**, 258; Gordh, T. In *The History of Anaesthesia*, edited by R. S. Atkinson and T. B. Boulton, Royal Society of Medicine, 1989, pp.441–442
7. Krawkow, N. F. *Arch. Exp. Path. Pharmak.*, 1908, Suppl. 317
8. Fischer, E. and von Mering, J. *Ther. d. Gegenw.*, 1903, **5**, 97
9. Bardet, D. *Bull. Gen. Therap.*, 1921, **1**, 27; Fredet, P. and Perlis, R. *Bull. et Mem. Soc. Nat. de Chir.*, 1924, **50**, 789
10. Noel, H. and Souttar, H. S. *Ann. Surg.*, 1913, **57**, 64

11. Bredenfeld, E. Z. *Exp. Path. Ther.*, 1916, **18**, 80
12. Bumm, R. *Klin. Wochenschr.*, 1927, **6**, 725
13. Zerfas, L. G. and McCallum, J. T. C. *J. Ind. Med. Assoc.*, 1929, **22**, 47
14. Fitch, R. H. *et al. Am. J. Surg.*, 1930, **NS9**, 110
15. Magill, I. W. *Lancet*, 1931, **1**, 74
16. Lundy, J. S. *Surg. Clin. North Am.*, 1931, **11**, 909
17. Kirschner, M. *Chirurg.*, 1929, **1**, 673; Macintosh, R. R. *et al. Lancet*, 1941, **2**, 10; Thornton, H. L. *et al. Anesthesiology*, 1945, **6**, 583
18. Weese, H. and Scharpff, W. *Dtsch. Med. Wochenschr.*, 1932, **58**, 1205
19. Jarman, R. and Abel, L. *Lancet*, 1933, **2**, 18
20. Tabern, D. L. and Volwiler, E. H. *J. Am. Chem. Soc.*, 1935, **57**, 1961
21. Pratt, T. W. *et al. Am. J. Surg.*, 1936, **31**, 464
22. Lundy, J. S. and Tovell, R. M. *North West Med.*, 1935, **33**, 308; Lundy, J. S. *Proc. Staff Meet. Mayo Clin.*, 1935, **10**, 536 (reprinted in 'Classical File', *Surv. Anesthesiol.*, 1958, **2**, 231); Corssen, G. In *Anaesthesia; Essays on its History*, edited by J. Rupreht *et al.*, Springer-Verlag, Berlin, 1985, p.88
23. Jarman, R. and Abel, L. *Lancet*, 1936, **1**, 422
24. Brodie, B. B. *et al. J. Pharmacol. Exp. Ther.*, 1950, **98**, 85 (reprinted in 'Classical File'. *Surv. Anesthesiol.*, 1965, **9**, 391)
25. Halford, F. J. *Anesthesiology*, 1943, **4**, 67; Bennetts, F. E. *Br. J. Anaesth.*, 1995, **75**, 366
26. Organe, G. S. W. *et al. Lancet*, 1938, **2**, 1170; see also Papper, E. M. The 50th anniversary of the use of thiopentone (editorial). *Anaesthesia*, 1984, **39**, 517; Dundee, J. W. Editorial. *Br. J. Anaesth.*, 1984, **56**, 211
27. See also Corssen, G. In *Anaesthesia; Essays on its History*, edited by J. Rupreht *et al.*, Springer-Verlag, Berlin, 1985, p.42
28. Lundy, J. S. *Minn. Med.*, 1926, **9**, 399
29. Chernish, S. M. *et al. Fed. Proc.*, 1956, **15**, 409
30. Stoelting, V. K. *Anesth. Analg. Curr. Res.*, 1957, **36**, 49
31. Dundee, J. W. and Moore, J. *Anaesthesia*, 1961, **16**, 50
32. See also Dundee, J. W. In *Anaesthesia, Essays on its History*, edited by J. Rupreht *et al.*, Springer-Verlag, Berlin, 1985, p.88
33. Ledingham, I. McA. and Watt, I. *Lancet*, 1983, **1**, 1270
34. Kay, B. and Rolly, G. *Acta Anaesthiol. Belg.*, 1977, **28**, 303
35. Rogers, K. M. *et al. Br. J. Anaesth.*, 1980, **52**, 407; Kay, B. and Stephenson, D. K. *Anaesthesia*, 1980, **35**, 1182; Rutter, D. V. *et al. Anaesthesia*, 1980, **35**, 1188; Kay, B. *Anaesthesia*, 1981, **36**, 863; Major, E. *et al. Br. J. Anaesth.*, 1981, **53**, 267
36. Dziewonski, K. and Sternbach, L. H. *Chem. Abst.*, 1936. **30**, 2971
37. Delay, J. *Psychopharmacological Frontiers*, Little, Brown & Co., Boston, 1959
38. De Castro, J. and Mundeleer, P. *Anesth. Anal. Paris*, 1959, **16**, 1022
39. Chen, G. *et al. J. Pharmacol. Exp. Ther.*, 1966, **152**, 332
40. Domino, E. F. *et al. Clin. Pharmacol. Ther.*, 1965, **6**. 279; Corssen, G. and Domino, E. F. *Anesth. Analg. Curr. Res.*, 1966, **45**, 29; Corssen, G. In *Anaesthesia; Essays on its History*, edited by J. Rupreht *et al.*, Springer-Verlag, Berlin, 1985, p.92; Boulton, T. B. Dissociative anesthesia. 'Classical File', *Surv. Anesthesiol.*, 1987, **31**, 62

41. Bion, J. F. *Anaesthesia*, 1984, **39**, 1023
42. See also White, P. F. *et al*. Ketamine; its pharmacology and therapeutic uses. *Anesthesiology* 1982, **56**, 119.
43. Powell, H., Morgan, M. and Sear, J. W., *Anaesthesia*, 1992, **47**, 287
44. Kenny, G. M. C. and White, M. In *Recent Advances in Anaesthesia and Analgesia 18*, edited by R. S. Atkinson and A. P. Adams, Churchill Livingstone, Edinburgh, 1994
45. Ellis, R. H. (ed.) *The Casebooks of Dr John Snow*, Wellcome Institute for the History of Medicine, 1995
46. Carman, J. A. *Anaesthesia*, 1968, **23**, 706
47. Holmes, T. *Brody*, T. Fischer Unwin, London, 1898
48. Brody, B. C. *Phil. Trans.*, 1811, **101**, 194; 1812, **102**, 205
49. Reprinted in 'Classical File', *Surv. Anesthesiol.*, 1978, **22**, 98; McDowall, G. *Anaesth. Intensive Care*, 1982, **10**, 4; Symposium on Charles Waterton. *Br. J. Anaesth.*, 1983, **55**, 221; Maltby, J. R. In *Anaesthesia; Essays on its History*, edited by J. Rupreht *et al.*, Springer-Verlag, Berlin, 1985; Edginton, B.W. *Charles Waterton: A Biography*, Lutterworth Press, Cambridge
50. Bernard, C. *C. R. Soc. Biol. Paris*, 1851, **2**, 195; *Leçon sur les Effets des Substances Toxiques et Médicamenteuses*, Baillière, Paris, 1851
51. Paton, A. *Practitioner*, 1979, **223**, 849
52. Sayer, L. A. *New York J. Med.*, 1858, **4**, 250
53. Fraser, T. R. *Trans. R. Soc. Edinburgh*, 1866/67, **24**, 715
54. Boehm, R. *Arch. Pharm.*, 1897, **235**, 660
55. Pal, J. *Zbl. Physiol.*, 1900, **14**, 255
56. Meltzer, S. J. and Auer, J. *J. Exp. Med.*, 1909, **2**, 622
57. Läwen, A. *Beitr. Klin. Chir.*, 1912, **80**, 168
58. Läwen, A. *Zbl. Chirurg.*, 1910, **37**, 708; *Dtsch. Zeit. Chir.*, 1911, **108**, 11
59. Dale, H. H. *J. Pharmacol. Exp. Ther.*, 1914, **6**, 147
60. Aeschlimann, J. A. and Reinart, M. *J. Pharmacol.*, 1931, **43**, 413
61. Cole, L. *Lancet*, 1934, **2**, 475
62. Dale, H. H. *Br. Med. J.*, 1934, **1**, 835
63. King, H. *J. Chem. Soc.*, 1935, **57**, 1381; *Nature*, 1935, **135**, 469
64. West, R. *Lancet*, 1936, **1**, 12
65. Dale, H. *et al. J. Physiol.*, 1936, **86**, 353
66. Bennett, A. E. *J.A.M.A.*, 1940, **114**, 322; Bennett, A. E. *et al. J.A.M.A.*, 1940, **114**, 1791; Bennett, A. E. *Am. J. Psychiatry*, 1941, **97**, 1014
67. Palmer, H. *J. Ment. Sci.*, 1946, **92**, 411
68. See also Griffith, H. R. and Johnson, E. *Anesthesiology*, 1942, **3**, 418; Giles, D. M. M. *Can. Anaesth. Soc. J.*, 1985, **32**, 570; 'Classical File', *Surv. Anesthesiol.*, 1985, **29**, 358; Seldon, T. H. *Anesth. Analg. (Cleve.)*, 1986, **65**, 1051 Bodman, R. and Gilles, D. *Harold Griffith*, Hannah Institute, 1992
69. Belcher, A. M. *Anesth. Analg. (Cleve.)*, 1977, **56**, 305
70. Griffith, H. R. and Johnson, G. E. *Anesthesiology*, 1942, **3**, 418–420 (reprinted in 'Classical File', *Surv. Anesthesiol.*, 1957, **1**, 174)
71. Wintersteiner, O. and Dutcher, J. D. *Science*, 1943, **97**, 467
72. Cullen, S. C. *Surgery*, 1943, **14**, 261
73. Seldon, T. H. *Anesth. Analg.*, 1986, **65**, 101

74. Waters, R. *Anesthesiology,* 1944, **5**, 618
75. Harroun, P. *et al. Anesthesiology,* 1946, **7**, 24
76. Mallinson, F. B. *Lancet,* 1945, **2**, 75
77. Gray, T. C. and Halton, J. A. *Proc. Roy. Soc. Med.,* 1946, **39**, 400 (reprinted in 'Classical File', *Surv. Anesthesiol.,* 1974, **18**, 500); Gray, T. C. *Br. J. Anaesth.,* 1983, **55**, 227
78. Bovet, D. *et al. C. R. Séances Acad. Sci.,* 1947, **225**, 74
79. Huguenard, P. and Boué, A. *C. R. Acad. Sci.,* 1948, **17**
80. Mushin, W. W. *et al. Lancet,* 1949, **1**, 726
81. Neff, W. B. *et al. Calif. Med.,* 1947, **66**, 67
82. Barlow, R. B. and Ing, H. R. *Nature,* 1948, **161**, 718; *Br. J. Pharmacol.,* 1948, **3**, 298 (reprinted in 'Classical File', *Surv. Anesthesiol.,* 1961, **5**, 213)
83. Paton, W. D. M. and Zaimis, E. J. *Nature,* 1948, **162**, 810
84. Bovet, D. *et al. R. C. 1st Sup. Sanot.,* 1949, **12**, 107
85. Castillo, J. C. and de Beer, E. J. *J. Pharmacol.,* 1950, **99**, 458 (reprinted in 'Classical File', *Surv. Anesthesiol.,* 1964, **8**, 42)
86. Hunt, R. and Taveau, R. de M. *Br. Med. J.,* 1906, **2**, 1788
87. von Dardel, O. and Thesleff, S. *Nord. Med.,* 1951, **46**, 1308; *Acta Chir. Scand.,* 1952, **103**, 321 (translated in 'Classical File', *Surv. Anesthesiol.,* 1967, **11**, 176)
88. Brücke, H. *et al. Wien. Klin. Wochenschr.,* 1951, **47**, 885; Mayerhofer, O. *Br. Med. J.,* 1952, **2**, 1332
89. Scurr, C. F. *Br. Med. J.,* 1951, **2**, 831
90. Grob, A. *et al. Bull. Johns Hopkins Hosp.,* 1949, **84**, 279
91. Churchill-Davidson, H. C. and Richardson, A. T. *Proc. Roy. Soc. Med.,* 1952, **45**, 179
92. Thesleff, S. *Acta Physiol. Scand.,* 1952, **25**, 348
93. Bourne, J. G. *et al. Lancet,* 1952, **1**, 1225
94. Forbat, A. *et al. Lancet,* 1953, **1**, 1067; Dorkin, H.R. *Med. Hist.,* 1982, **26**, 145
95. Beecher, H. K. and Todd, D. P. *Ann. Surg.,* 1954, **140**, 2 (reprinted in 'Classical File', *Surv. Anesthesiol.,* 1971, **15**, 394, 496)
96. Paton, W. D. M. *Br. J. Anaesth.,* 1956, **28**, 470
97. Pridgen, J. E. *Surgery,* 1956, **40**, 571
98. Bernauer, K. *et al. Helv. Chim. Acta,* 1958, **41**, 2293
99. Hugin, W. and Kissling, P. *Schweiz. Med. Wochenschr.,* 1961, **91**, 445; Seegar, R. *et al. Anaesthesist,* 1962, **11**, 37; Lund, L. and Stovner, J. *Acta Anaesthesiol. Scand.,* 1962, **6**, 85
100. Baird, W. L. M. and Reid, A. M. *Br. J. Anaesth.,* 1967, **39**, 775 (reprinted in 'Classical File', *Surv. Anesthesiol.,* 1981, **25**, 133); Crul, J. F. *Proc. 4th World Congr. Anaesth.,* Excerpta Medica, Amsterdam, 1968, p.418
101. Burkett, W. R. and Bonta, K. L. *Fed. Proc.,* 1966, **25**, 718
102. Everett, A. J. *et al. J. Chem. Soc.,* 1970, Sect. D, Chem. Commun., 1020
103. Tunstall, M. E. *Br. Med. J.,* 1977, **1**, 1321
104. Durant, N. N. *et al. J. Pharm. Pharmacol.,* 1979, **31**, 831; Crul, J. F. and Booij, L. H. D. J. *Br. J. Anaesth.,* 1980, **52**, 495

105. Stenlake, J. B. In *Advances in Pharmacology and Therapeutics*, edited by J. P. Stoclet, Pergamon, Oxford, 1980; Hughes, R. and Chapple, D. J. *Br. J. Anaesth.*, 1980, **52**, 238P

106. Savarese, J. J. *et al. Anesthesiology*, 1988, **68**, 723; Kreig, N. and Crul, J. F. *et al. Br. J. Anaesth.*, 1980, **52**, 783; Hughes, R. and Chapple, D. J. *Br. J. Anaesth.*, 1981, **53**, 31; Payne, J. P. and Hughes, R. *Br. J. Anaesth.*, 1981, **53**, 45

107. Booij, L. H. D. J. and Knape, H. T. A. *Anaesthesia*, 1991, **46**, 341

108. Elsholtz, J.S. *Clysmatica Nova 1665*. Facsimile Ed, Matsuki, A. Iwanimi Book Service Center, Tokyo, 1995 with English translation by Ward, M.

8
Opioids and other drugs used during anaesthesia

Opioids

The opioids[1] have been very commonly used by anaesthetists from the beginning of the speciality. Crude opium was available in Asia two millennia before the discovery of modern anaesthesia, and was used through the Middle Ages in Europe as the preparation 'laudanum'. The development and use of opioids for the relief of human suffering in the nineteenth and twentieth centuries has been one of the humanitarian success stories of modern medicine. The first step was the isolation of **morphine** from opium by Freidrich Seturner in 1803.[2] It was first given hypodermically using a vaccination lancet, by G. V. Lafargue of St. Emilion in 1836.[3]

Diamorphine was synthesized by Beckett and Wright in 1875.[4] This marked the first chemical manipulation of natural opioids for production of analgesics. Diamorphine (heroin) was prepared at St. Mary's Hospital, London, in 1898, and was intended for control of morphine addicts. The tragedy was that it caused more addiction than morphine! **Papaveretum (Omnopon)** was prepared in 1909 by Hermann Sahli (1856–1933) of Berne[5] as a pharmaceutically standardized preparation of crude opium. It was marketed in Germany as Pantopon. Later, as Omnopon,[6] it became popular in the UK, as it was one of the first opiates to become available in solution in ampoules.

The next step was the production of a completely synthetic opioid. **Pethidine** was synthesized in 1939 by Schaumann and Eisleb in Germany during a search for an atropine substitute.[7] It was first used in premedication by Schlungbaum[8] and in the USA in 1943.[9] Later during World War II, **methadone** was also developed in Germany, and was originally named 'dolfine' in honour of *Adolf* Hitler.

Fentanyl and **alfentanil** were produced in 1962 by Janssen and co-workers.[10] The rapid onset and short duration of action of this group of drugs made them very useful in the practice of anaesthesia. It was an important development because they fitted the needs of operative analgesia very well. Further synthetic agents similar to these were developed for veterinary practice.

Opioid peptides were discovered in 1979 by Goldstein *et al.*,[11] but they have not yet made a mark on clinical anaesthesia. **Sufentanil** followed soon after this.[12]

An important step in the history of analgesia was taken when Pohl demonstrated the reversal of opiate respiratory depression by N-allyl-norcodeine.[13] Levallorphan was discovered in the 1940s but was not totally satisfactory. N-allyl-normorphine (**nalorphine**) followed in the 1950s, with a better antagonist profile. The search for a pure opiate antagonist resulted in the appearance of **naloxone** in 1971[14] and subsequently the long-acting nalmefine.

Opioid receptors

Keats and Telford, investigating nalorphine in 1956,[15] found evidence of receptors for opioids, a concept which was developed by Martin *et al.* in 1976,[16] who proposed mu (analgesia); kappa (sedation) and delta (respiratory depression) receptor subtypes. The mu receptors were later subdivided into mu_1 (analgesia) and mu_2 (respiratory depression). Pleuvry[17] proposed that adrenergic receptor occupation could influence the analgesic action of opioids, which led directly to the alpha-1 and alpha-2 adrenergic agonist clonidine being developed for potentiation of opioid analgesia without augmentation of respiratory depression. The alpha-2 agonist, dexmedetomidine was then investigated by Bloor *et al.* for the same purpose.[18] This drug has already found a place in veterinary anaesthesia.

Epidural and spinal opioids were made possible in 1976 when Yaksh and Rudy[19] demonstrated their direct action on the spinal cord. The exact site of action, the substantia gelatinosa, was uncovered by Snyder the following year.[20] The clinical use of epidural morphine followed the classic paper by Behar *et al.* in 1979.[21]

Some ancillary drugs

The last quarter of the twentieth century has witnessed an explosion in the number of ancillary drugs used for various purposes during the course of anaesthesia. These, in the hands of anaesthetists and surgeons, have added a dimension of safety for the sick surgical patient.

Heparin was first discovered in 1916 by a medical student in Baltimore[22] and remains in use 80 years later as first-choice anticoagulant for extracorporeal bypass and for prophylaxis for deep vein thrombosis.

The adrenal glands had been described by Bartholomaeus in 1563 and modern knowledge of adrenal physiology started with the description by Thomas Addison (1793–1860) of London in 1855 of the disease of hypoadrenalism which bears his name. **Adrenaline** itself was isolated by George Oliver (1841–1915), a practitioner in Harrogate, and J. J. Abel of the Johns Hopkins Hospital and Sir Edward Schäfer (1850–1935) in 1894[23] from the adrenal medulla, who showed that it contained a pressor agent. It was produced in crystalline form by Takamine (1854–1922)[24] (who determined its constitution and patented it under the name of 'adrenaline')[25] and Aldrich,[26] independently, in 1901. It was the first hormone to be synthesized. Friedrich Stolz (1860–1936) also produced it in 1904.[27] Adrenaline remains first-line treatment for circulatory support, resuscitation, treatment of anaphylaxis, severe bronchospasm, and for producing local vasoconstriction.

The word 'hormone' (Greek = to set in motion) was introduced by E. H. Starling (1866–1927) of London in 1905).[28]

The role of **noradrenaline** in the transmission of nerve impulses was described by Elliott in 1905 and proved by Otto Loewi (1873–1961) of Berlin, in 1921.[29] The properties of racemic noradrenaline were described by George Barger (1878–1939) and Henry Hallett Dale (1875–1968) in 1910.[30]

The alpha and beta agonist **ephedrine** was introduced into Western medicine in 1924 by Chen and Schmidt,[31] and its use was soon espoused by anaesthetists for cardiovacular support in spinal analgesia. This active principle of ma huang, a Chinese plant, had been isolated in 1885 by Yamanash and named by N. Nagai (1844–1929) in 1887.[32] It was later manufactured synthetically. Its adrenaline-like properties were described by Japanese pharmacologists in 1917.[33] It continues as one of the most-used drugs for raising arterial pressure during anaesthesia, especially spinal or extradural anaesthesia, with a rapid yet controlled action.

Of the other vasoconstrictors, **methoxamine hydrochloride** was synthesized in 1942,[34] and was first used to maintain blood pressure in spinal analgesia in 1950. **Phenylephrine hydrochloride** was described in 1910 by Barger and Dale,[35] and later by Kuschinsky and Oberdisse.[36] It was first used as a pressor agent in spinal analgesia in 1938.[37]

Doxapram hydrochloride had its debut in 1962,[38] and is still a useful postoperative respiratory stimulant.

References

1. Verner, I.R., *Current Anaesthesia and Critical Care*, 1994, **5**, 178–182
2. Seturner, F.W.A. *J.Pharm.fur Aertze und Apoth.Chem. Leipzig*, 1806, **14**, 17

3. Lafargue, G.V. *C. R. Acad. Sci. Paris*, 1836, **2**, 397
4. Beckett, L. and Wright, M., *J. Chem. Soc.*, 1875, **28**, 312
5. Sahli, H. *Ther. Mh. Halbruch*, 1909, **23**, 1
6. Leipoldt, C.L. *Lancet*, 1911, **1**, 368; Kerri Szanto, M. *Can. Anaesth. Soc. J.*, 1974, **23**, 239
7. Schaumann, O. and Eisleb, O., *Dtsch. Med. Wochenschr.*, 1939, **65**, 967
8. Schlungbaum, H. *Med. Klin.*, 1939, **35**, 1259
9. Rovenstine, E.A. and Battermann, R.I. *Anesthesiology*, 1943, **4**, 126
10. Janssen, P.A.J. *Br. J. Anaesth.* 1962, **34**, 260–268
11. Goldstein, A., Tachibana, S., Lowney, L.I. *et al. Proc. Natl Acad. Sci. USA*, 1979, **76**, 6666–6670
12. Bovill, J.G., Sebel, P.S., Blackburn, C.L. *et al. Anesthesiology*, 1984, **61**, 502–506
13. Pohl, J. *Z.Exp.Path.Ther.*, 1915, **17**, 370–382
14. Clark, R.B. *J.Arkansas Med. Soc.*, 1971, **68**, 128
15. Keats, A.S. and Telford, J. *J. Pharmacol. Exp. Ther.*, 1956, **117**, 190
16. Martin, W.R., Eades, C.G., Thompson, J.A. *et al. J. Pharmacol. Exp. Ther.* 1976, **197**, 517–532
17. Pleuvry, B.J. *Br. J. Anaesth.*, 1983, **55**, 143S–146S
18. Bloor, B.C., Raybould, D., Shurtliffe, M. *et al. Anesthesiology*, 1988, **69**, A614
19. Yaksh, T.L. and Rudy, T.A. *Science*, 1976, **192**, 1357–1358
20. Snyder, S.H. Opiate receptors in the brain. *N. Engl. J. Med.*, 1977, **296**, 266–271
21. Behar, M., Magori F., Olshwang D. and Davidson J.T. *Lancet*, 1979, **1**, 527–530
22. McLean, J. *Am. J. Physiol.*, 1916, **41**, 250
23. Oliver, G. and Schäfer, E.A. *J. Physiol.*, 1895, **18**, 230
24. Takamine, J. *Therapeutic. Gaz.* 1901, **27**, 221
25. Takamine, J. *Am. J. Pharmacol.*, 1901, **73**, 523
26. Aldrich, T.B. *Am. J. Physiol.* 1901, **5**, 457
27. Stolz, F. *Berl. Chem. Ges.*, 1904, **37**, 4149
28. Starling, E.H. *Lancet*, 1905, **2**, 339
29. Loewi, O. *Pflugers Arch.*, 1921, **189**, 239
30. Barger, G. and Dale, H.H. *J. Physiol.*, 1910, **41**, 19
31. Chen, K.K. and Schmidt, C.F. *J. Pharmacol. Exp. Ther.*, 1924, **24**, 339
32. Nagai, N. *Pharm. Zeit.*, 1887, **32**, 7000
33. Amatsu, H. and Kubota, S. *Kyoto Igâai Zasski*, 1917, **14**, 77
34. Baltzly, R. and Buck, J.S. *J. Am. Chem. Soc.*, 1942, **64**, 3040
35. Barger, G. and Dale, H.H. *J. Physiol.* 1910, **41**, 19
36. Kuschinsky, G. and Oberdisse, K. *Arch. Exp. Path. Pharmak.*, 1931, **162**, 46
37. Lorhan, P.H. and Oliverio, R.M. *Curr. Res.. Anesth. Analg.*, 1938, **17**, 44
38. Dundee, J.W. *et al. Br. J. Pharmacol.*, 1973, **48**, 326P

9
Intubation of the trachea

Tracheal intubation for resuscitation

Tracheal insufflation in animals was described by Andreas Vesalius (1514–64) of Padua in 1543,[1] and by Robert Hooke (1635–1703) in 1667.[2] The end of the eighteenth century produced a flurry of research and publications of intubation of the trachea (triggered by the humanitarian concern for the resuscitation of the drowned) by a few individuals in Britain and the Netherlands. The historical significance of this is that it was the publications of a very few visionaries which alerted widespread public interest in the subject. Cogan published the Transactions of the Amsterdam Society for the Recovery of Drowned Persons in 1773, and formed a similar society in England with Hawes in 1774, which became the Royal Humane Society in 1787. Their work showed that intubation was more efficient than mouth-to-mouth ventilation!

In 1776, John Hunter described a metal tracheal tube,[3] and C. Kite from Gravesend described oral and nasal intubation for resuscitation of the apparently drowned in 1788.[4] James Curry described several different metal endotracheal tubes in 1792.[5] These techniques were surveyed by Danish workers, J. D. Herholt and C. G. Rafn, in 1796.[6]

Pierre Joseph Desault (1744–95) and his pupil Marie F.-X. Bichat (1771–1802) were early intubators for laryngeal obstruction. In 1827 Leroy showed that pneumothorax may result from high lung inflation pressures.[7] John Snow used a tracheal catheter to resuscitate a newborn baby,[8] although he gives no technical details in his casebooks.

eal intubation for inhalation anaesthesia

All the work noted above was directed at either resuscitation or the relief of upper airway obstruction. Passage of a tube or catheter into the trachea was practised for the attempted resuscitation of the earliest anaesthetic casualties from 1848. It was a significant advance to contemplate deliberately instrumenting the trachea for the sole pupose of administering anaesthetic vapours. John Snow made this historical leap by intubating animals via a tracheotomy in 1852. Friederich Trendelenburg (1844–1924) of Rostock used the method in man in 1871 while he was a surgical assistant to Langenbeck in Berlin. He used it for operations on the mouth, and after performing a tracheotomy, occluded the trachea by an inflatable cuff, using a tube he had described in 1869.[9]

It had been assumed that a tube passing through the larynx would not be tolerated, but William MacEwen (1847–1924)* of Glasgow decided, in 1878, to try to avoid the tracheotomy that was otherwise inevitable. After practising on the cadaver, he passed a flexible metal tube from the mouth into the trachea, using his fingers as a guide in a conscious patient.[11] Through this tube he gave chloroform and air for removal of a carcinoma of the base of the tongue. A sponge was packed round the superior laryngeal aperture

---

* Sir William MacEwen (1847–1924)[10]

Born in Rothesay in the Isle of Bute, Scotland, on 22 June 1847, the youngest of 12 children and son of a sea captain, just 7 months after Simpson's introduction of chloroform. Medical student at the University of Glasgow, where he qualified in 1869 and proceeded to the MD degree 3 years later. While the Regius Professor of Surgery, Joseph Lister, was developing his system of antiseptic surgery, MacEwen became his dresser. This association with the great man had a profound effect on MacEwen's subsequent professional development. Following resident appointments in the Royal Infirmary, he was appointed Medical Superintendent of the Belvedere Fever Hospital, where he had the harrowing experience of treating patients suffering from respiratory obstruction due to laryngeal diphtheria, an experience which led him to his great discovery of oral laryngeal intubation.

Leaving the Fever Hospital, he went into general practice and became a parochial medical officer. Gradually his interests centred on surgery, and he obtained appointments at both the Glasgow Royal Infirmary and Western Infirmary, culminating in his nomination to the Chair as Regius Professor of Surgery in the University of Glasgow in 1877, a post he was to fill with great distinction for the next 15 years. Invited to become the first Professor of Surgery at the new Johns Hopkins Hospital in Baltimore, but refused it, the post going to William Stewart Halsted. On the accession of King Edward VII in 1902, MacEwan was knighted. Became President of the British Medical Association in 1922 and of the International College of Surgeons when it met in London the following year.

A tall, handsome man, and an impressive personality who tolerated fools badly, he went his own way. His numerous surgical contributions included the diagnosis and treatment of cerebral abscess, surgery of the brain, spine, chest and bones. An early exponent of aseptic surgery in which sterilization of instrument and dressings was carried out by heat. In addition to his great technical advances, MacEwen paid constant attention to teaching his students the rudiments of safe anaesthesia, a form of tuition uncommon at that time. Remained a great believer in chloroform anaesthesia. Became a Surgeon Rear-Admiral and Consultant to the Royal Navy in Scotland in 1914.

to protect the lungs from contamination. He had previously used rubber and gum elastic catheters for the relief of obstruction in laryngeal diphtheria.

These early attempts were often made to prevent aspiration pneumonia in surgery of the upper air passages. Karl Maydl (1853–1903) of Prague employed the metal tube of J. P. O'Dwyer (1841–98) of Cleveland[12] (designed for the treatment of laryngeal diphtheria, and introduced using special curved forceps) during such surgery in 1893.[13] Franz Kuhn of Kassel (1866–1929)[14] extended and developed the technique in 1901 by using a flexible metal tube introduced on a curved guide through the mouth, palpating the epiglottis with the fingers of his left hand. His preference was for inhalation anaesthesia, the patient breathing to and fro through the tube.[15]

Tracheal intubation for insufflation anaesthesia

In 1907, Barthélemy and Dufour of Nancy, France, blew chloroform vapour and air from a Vernon Harcourt (1834–1919) inhaler[16] through a rubber catheter, guided into the trachea by touch – the first use of insufflation endotracheal anaesthesia.[17] Samuel James Meltzer (1851–1920) and his son-in-law John Auer (1875–1948), physiologists at the Rockefeller Institute, New York City, furthered insufflation endotracheal anaesthesia in animals in 1909.[18] They blew anaesthetic vapour through a narrow tube placed near the carina, the gases returning either through a second tube or around the insufflation tube. The neurosurgeon Charles Albert Elsberg (1871–1948) of New York and others[19] applied the technique to man in the same year, while in 1912 Robert Kelly (1879–1944) of Liverpool brought the method to Britain.[20]

The establishment of tracheal intubation

Largely as a result of their experiences after World War I as anaesthetists for Sir Harold Gillies, the plastic surgeon at the Queen's Hospital for Facial and Jaw Injuries at Sidcup, Kent (1919), Edgar Stanley Rowbotham (1890–1979) and Ivan Whiteside Magill[21] (1888–1986) (Figure 9.1) used first insufflation through one (later two) narrow gum-elastic tubes passed via a laryngoscope (one insufflating warm ether vapour from a Shipway apparatus[22] with an electric motor, the other carrying it away), and then inhalation endotracheal methods, breathing in and out through a single tube.[23]

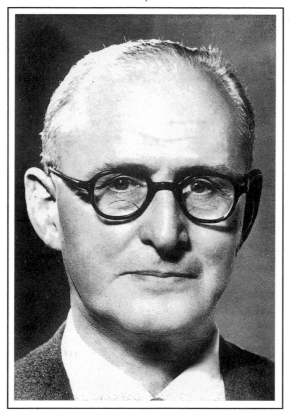

Figure 9.1 Sir Ivan Whiteside Magill (1888–1986)[32]

Born in Larne, Northern Ireland. Attended the local grammar school and then became a medical student at Queen's University, Belfast, qualifying in 1913. Became a house surgeon at the Stanley Hospital in Liverpool, and with the outbreak of World War I joined the RAMC and served with the Irish Guards at the battle of Loos. When peace came again, Magill was posted to the Queen's Hospital in Sidcup, Kent. With his colleague, Stanley Rowbotham (1890–1979), aged 32, neither of whom was at that time an experienced anaesthetist, they soon found themselves responsible for giving anaesthetics for reconstructive operations on the face and jaws in wounded soldiers, under the care of Harold Gillies, later to become a world famous pioneer of plastic surgery. Here, after trial and error, they became among the first workers to develop tracheal intubation. They were also among the first to develop the technique of nasotracheal intubation by the so-called blind method. The Magill tubes were eventually to become indispensable to all anaesthetists.

When the work at the unit in Sidcup decreased, Magill decided to devote his professional life to the administration of anaesthetics and was soon elected to the staffs of various hospitals in London. Eventually he chose the Westminster Hospital and the Brompton Hospital for Diseases of the Chest as his main bases. In addition, his skill and his personality enabled him to acquire a large private practice in London and beyond. He was a man of great practical ingenuity and over the years originated or developed many new pieces of equipment and refinements of technique for the safety of his patients and the convenience of his surgeons. Among these must be mentioned his laryngoscope and laryngeal forceps, and the 'Magill attachment', a simple combination of a breathing tube, reservoir bag and expiratory valve, used for spontaneous respiration (Mapleson A circuit), which featured on all anaesthetic machines in the UK for over 50 years. Developed methods of administering anaesthetics in thoracic surgery, employing endobronchial tubes and bronchus blockers for the control of pulmonary secretions, and these techniques for the production of one-lung anaesthesia greatly contributed to the development of thoracic surgery in the 1920s and 1930s.

Took a leading part in organizing the Association of Anaesthetists of Great Britain and Ireland in 1932; in instituting an examination for the Diploma in Anaesthetics (the first such examination in 1935); and in persuading the Royal College of Surgeons of England to found a Faculty of Anaesthetists in 1947. His understanding of medical history which led to this simple initiative cannot be overestimated. His great experience and his reputation as a safe and skilled clinical anaesthetist resulted in his being asked to employ his abilities on a large number of very distinguished patients, including many members of the British and other royal families when they required surgical treatment. He received a very large number of honours and medals including a knighthood (the KCVO) awarded personally by the Queen in 1960, the FRCS (Eng), the honorary FFARCS, the DSc of his old University, the Henry Hill Hickman Medal from the Royal Society of Medicine, and many others. For 50 years he was the doyen of British anaesthetists and his name was known world-wide. Tracheal intubation is the *sine qua non* of safe anaesthesia in many operations and this is largely due to the work of Ivan Magill and his colleague Stanley Rowbotham. In the 1920s when Ivan Magill's career began, anaesthesia was a little regarded speciality and those who practised it exclusively attracted little esteem from their colleagues. Magill lived to see it achieve parity with other specialities, a change in which he took a leading part because of his clinical pre-eminence and his international reputation.

The first blind nasal intubation was performed by Rowbotham.[24] Magill published his results of blind nasal intubation with a wide-bore rubber tube during the years following 1928.[25] This technique revolutionized the use of tracheal tubes in anaesthesia because it was quick, accurate, and gained early control of the airway, with the safety which that provided. Inflatable cuffs had been used for many years (e.g. Dorrance[26]), but were reintroduced by Arthur E. Guedel and Ralph Milton Waters in 1928.[27] A pilot balloon had been described in 1893 by Victor Eisenmenger (1864–1932),[28] by A. W. Green in 1906[29] and was reintroduced by C. Langton Hewer in 1939.[30]

While the methods of Magill and Rowbotham earned for them the support and approval of the surgeons with whom they worked, many other surgeons discouraged the use of intubation, partly because of the possibility of tissue damage and partly due to conservatism. It took many years before intubation was accepted by all anaesthetists. Those who learnt how to perform blind nasal intubation soon realized its great advantages, especially the fact that it would enable a patient to be taken to the level of anaesthesia necessary for a laparotomy very quickly with ether (then the commonly used agent), greatly reducing the time for induction. In addition, intubation provided a clear airway, prevented laryngeal spasm and enabled the lungs to be protected against aspiration of foreign material. Only when muscle relaxants became available was it possible to perform oral intubation rapidly, as direct laryngoscopy had previously needed a deep plane of inhalational anaesthesia. The use of muscle relaxants to facilitate intubation in the UK was pioneered by Bourne.[31] This turning point in anaesthesia was long overdue and credit is due to Bourne for convincing the postwar generation of anaesthetists of the value of relaxants for this purpose.

Endotracheal tubes

Traditional tubes for either nasal or oral intubation were Magill tubes of mineralized rubber. The red colour was due to the preservative. Oral tubes had thicker walls than nasal ones. The angled Oxford tube was thicker in the pharyngeal part and thinner in the tracheal part. Polyvinyl chloride (PVC) replaced these progressively from the 1950s. The toxicity of the PVC was tested by implantation in rabbit muscle (IT = 'implantation tested') or by cell culture. Z79 was the committee in the USA that originally approved anaesthetic equipment (1956). RAE preformed tubes (Wallace H. Ring, John C. Adair, Richard A. Elwyn, Salt Lake City anaesthetists) were developed in the 1980s.

Laryngoscopy and laryngoscopes

Indirect laryngoscopy with a mirror was pioneered by M. Garcia (1805–1906), a teacher of singing in London,[33] and became widely used for diagnostic purposes. Direct laryngoscopy was pioneered in 1895 by Alfred Kirstein (1863–1922) of Berlin[34] who called his instrument an 'autoscope'. The original bronchoscopist, Gustav Killian (1860–1921) of Freiburg,[35] developed this in 1912. Chevalier Jackson (1865–1958) of Philadelphia did his first bronchoscopy in 1899, and published a book on the subject in 1907[36] which also popularized direct laryngoscopy.

Jackson himself designed a laryngoscope[37] which was later modified by Magill[38] in 1926, Paluel J. Flagg (1886–1970) of New York,[39] R. A. Miller[40] and Robert Reynolds Macintosh of Oxford (1897–1989)[41] (Figure 9.2) in 1932. Magill's laryngoscope was modelled on that of William Hill[42], laryngologist to St. Mary's Hospital,

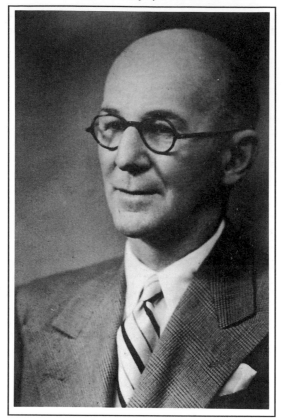

Figure 9.2 Sir Robert Reynolds Macintosh (1897–1989)[45]

Born at Timaru, New Zealand, travelled to Britain when World War I broke out, and joined the Royal Flying Corps, becoming a prisoner of war. Qualified in medicine from Guy's Hospital in 1924 and after abandoning a career in surgery became a successful dental anaesthetist in London with the 'Mayfair Gas Company', who carried their entire apparatus from surgery to surgery in the boot of a car. In 1937 he moved to Oxford to become the first Nuffield Professor of Anaesthetics in the University, the first such chair in Europe. Built up a renowned department in Oxford, undertaking clinical work, teaching and the development of anaesthetic apparatus. Secured the appointment of anaesthetic sisters and nurses, wrote textbooks noted for their clarity and encouraged the practice of regional analgesia. *Essentials of General Anaesthesia*, which he wrote with Dr Freda Bannister, was the first anaesthetic book to be published by Blackwell Scientific Publications Ltd, in 1941. Was first and foremost a clinical anaesthetist and his name became associated with many practical pieces of equipment, the most famous being the Macintosh laryngoscope. Macintosh had an enormous and wordwide influence on the evolution of anaesthesia and had exceptional skill in choosing the right people for the right jobs. Travelled to many countries, including the underdeveloped ones, and his work was recognized by the bestowal of honorary degrees from Universities in Argentina, France and Poland.

Was made an Honorary Fellow of the Faculties of Anaesthetists in England, Ireland and Australia and an Honorary Doctor of Science in the University of Wales. Knighted in 1955.

London. The light was originally powered from the electric mains, but is now supplied from a 3–volt battery in the handle or by a fibreoptic cable. The Macintosh instrument's blade was shorter, curved and Z-shaped on cross-section. Its tip entered the vallecula, lifted the base of the tongue, and with it the epiglottis, so that the cords could be visualized. It did not generate so much laryngeal spasm. It was produced by Charles King and later by the Penlon company. It was an immediate success and has continued to be so. One reason for this is that it can be used in lighter planes of anaesthesia, as it does not stimulate the posterior surface of the epiglottis. Macintosh also developed the laryngeal forceps which bear his name, used for directing nasal tubes under direct vision into the larynx.

The polio laryngoscope was designed for use on patients in iron-lung respirators; its Macintosh-type blade made an angle of approximately 135° with the handle.[43] The Bullard intubating laryngoscope was developed for situations where the neck was immobile and mouth opening restricted. It had fibreoptics, suction and intubation channels, and was made in adult and paediatric versions.[44]

Topical analgesia for intubation

Cocaine was first used to suppress the laryngeal reflex in general anaesthesia by Rosenberg in 1895[46] and by Magill, to aid intubation, in 1928.[47] Many sprays have been described for applying local anaesthetic to the larynx, e.g. the Forrester,[48] later supplanted by metered-dose aerosols. Lignocaine is now generally preferred because of its lower toxicity.

The laryngeal mask airway[49]

The invention of the laryngeal mask airway (Figure 9.3) completed a cycle in the history of anaesthesia, being developed by a determined individual anaesthetist, (A.Brain) – a remarkable achievement in the late twentieth century! It was then manufactured by an equipment company, Colgate Medical. This inventive spirit was the driving force of the early days of anaesthesia, although in the nineteenth century it was unencumbered by bureaucratic restric-

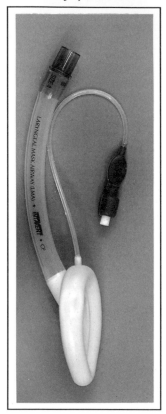

Figure 9.3   Laryngeal mask airway

tions. Although small masks had been tried in the pharynx before, and rejected, the improved materials and design of the laryngeal mask airway, coupled with the timely arrival of propofol, which suppressed pharyngeal and laryngeal reflexes, allowed a successful outcome.

The laryngeal mask did not necessarily prevent aspiration, but was often easy to insert in patients who were very difficult to intubate.[50] It proved to be extremely convenient and safe. Several versions were developed for various special functions, including intermittent positive pressure ventilation, and resuscitation.

The **oesophageal obturator airway** was developed for use in resuscitation, mainly outside the hospital environment.[51] The **oesophageal gastric tube airway** was passed into the oesophagus and its cuff inflated with about 35 ml of air. It displaced the larynx forward and provided an airway. Again, it was designed for resuscitation[52] but did not find wide acceptance.

See also McCartney, C. and Wilkinson, D.J. *Curr. Anaesth. Crit. Care*, 1995, **6**, 54–58; Baniji, A. *Curr. Anaesth Crit.Care*, 1996, **7**, 44–48.

References

1. *De Fabrica Humani Corporis*, 1543; see also Wedley, J.R. *Br. J. Clin. Equip.*, 1979, **4**, 49
2. Hooke, R. An account of an experiment made by M. Hook of preserving animals alive by blowing through their lungs with bellows. *Phil. Trans. Roy. Soc.*, 1667, **2**
3. Hunter, J. *Proposals for the recovery of persons apparently drowned*, London 1776
4. Kite, C. *An Essay on the recovery of the apparently dead*, C.Dilley in the Poultry, London, 1788; Davison, M.H.A. *Br. J. Anaesth.*, 1951, **23**, 238
5. Curry, J. *Observations on apparent death from drowning, suffocation etc. with an account of the means to be employed for recovery*, Northampton, 1792
6. Herholdt, J.D. and Rafn, C.G. *An attempt at an historical survey of life-saving measures for drowned persons, and information of the best means by which they can be brought back to life*, Tikiob, Copenhagen, 1796
7. Leroy, J. Recherches sur l'asphyxie. *J. Physiol. Exp. Pathol.*, 1827, **7**, 45–64; *ibid.*, 1828, **8**, 97–135
8. Ellis, R.H. (ed.) *The Casebooks of Dr John Snow*, Wellcome Institute for the History of Medicine, 1995, p.30
9. Trendelenburg, F. *Arch. Klin. Chir.*, 1871, **12**, 121
10. See also Keys, T.E. *Anesth. Analg. Curr. Res.*, 1974, **53**, 537; James C.D.T. *Anaesthesia*, 1974, **29**, 743; Bowman, A.K. *The Life and Teaching of Sir William MacEwan*, W. Hodge and Co., London 1942; Wakeley, C. (ed.) *Great Teachers of Surgery in the Past*, Wright, Bristol, 1969
11. MacEwen, W. *Glas. Med. J.*, 1879, **2**, 72; *Br. Med. J.*, 1880, **2**, 122 (reprinted in 'Classical File', *Surv. Anesthesiol.*, 1969, **13**, 105)
12. O'Dwyer, J. *Med. Rec.*, 1887, **32**, 557
13. Maydl, K. *Wien. Med. Wochenschr.*, 1893, **43**, 102
14. Kuhn, F. *Die perorale intubation* S. Karger, Berlin, 1911; Zinganell, K. *Anaesthesist* 1974, **23**, 308; Sweeney, B. *Anaesthesia*, 1985, **40**, 1000–1005
15. Kuhn, F. *Zbl. Chir.*, 1901, **28**, 1281
16. Harcourt, V. *Br. Med. J.*, 18 July, 1903, **2**, 162
17. Barthélemy and Dufour, *Presse Méd.*, 1907, **15**, 475
18. Meltzer, S.J. and Auer, J. Continuous respiration without respiratory movements. *J. Exp. Med.*, 1909, **11**, 622–625
19. Elsberg, C.A. *N. Y. Med. Rec.*, 1910, **77**, 493; *Ann. Surg.*, 1910, **52**, 23; Intratracheal insufflation anaesthesia, its value in thoratic and general surgery. *New York State J. Med.*, 1912, **12**(1), 524–528

20. Kelly, R.E. *Br. Med. J.*, 1912, **2**, 617, 1121
21. Magill, I.W. *Lancet*, 1923, **2**, 228; *Anaesthesia*, 1975, **30**, 476; Condon, H.A. and Gilchrist, E. *Anaesthesia*, 1986, **41**, 46
22. Shipway, F. *Lancet*, 1916, **1**, 70
23. Rowbotham, E.S. and Magill, I.W. *Proc. Roy. Soc. Med.*, 1921, **14**, 17; Magill, I.W. *Proc. Roy. Soc. Med.*, 1929, **22**, 83 (reprinted in 'Classical File', *Surv. Anesthesiol.*, 1978, **33**, 580)
24. Rowbotham, E.S. *Br. Med. J.* 1920. **2**, 590
25. Magill, I.W. *Brt. Med. J.* 1930, **2**, 817
26. Dorrance, G.M. *Surg. Gynecol. Obstet.* 1910, **11**, 160
27. Guedel, A.E. and Waters, R.M. *Curr. Res. Anesth. Analg.*, 1928, **7**, 238 (reprinted in 'Classical File', *Surv. Anesthesiol.*, 1984, **28**, 71)
28. Eisenmenger, V. *Wien. Med. Wochenschr.*, 1893, **43**, 199
29. Green, N.W. *Surg. Gynecol. Obstet.*, 1906, **2**, 512
30. Hewer, C.L. *Recent Advances in Anaesthesia and Analgesia*, 3rd edn, Churchill, London, 1939, p.115
31. Bourne, J.G. *Br. Med. J.*, 1947, **2**, 654
32. See also Gillespie, N.A. (1943) In *Endotracheal Anesthesia*, 2nd edn, edited by B. J. Bamforth and K. L. Siebeckar, University of Wisconsin Press, 1943; Waters, R.M. and Guedel, A.E. Endotracheal anaesthesia: its historical development. *Anesth. Analg. Curr. Res.*, 1933, **12**, 196 (reprinted in 'Classical File', *Surv. Anesthesiol.*, 1984, **28**, 76); Bowes, J.B. and Zorab, J.S.M. Sir Ivan Magill's contributions to anaesthesia. In *Anaesthesia: Essays on its History*, edited by J. Rupreht et al., Springer-Verlag, Heidelberg, 1985, p.13; Edridge, A.W. *Anaesthesia*, 1987, **42**, 231–233
33. Garcia, M. *Proc. Roy. Soc. Lond.*, 1855, **7**, 399
34. Kirstein, A. *Allg. Med. ZentZtg*, 1895, **34**, 110; *Lancet*, 1895, **1**, 1132; *Berlin Klin.Wschr*, 1895, **32**, 476–478; Hirsch, N.P. *et al. Anaesthesia*, 1986, **41**, 42; McCartney, C. and Wilkinson, D.J. *Current Anaesthesia and Critical Care*, 1995, **6**, 54–58
35. Zollner, F. *Arch. Otolaryngol*, 1965, **82**, 656
36. Jackson, C. *Tracheobronchoscopy, Esophagoscopy and Gastroscopy*, Mosby, St Louis, 1907
37. Jackson, C. *Surg. Gynecol. Obstet.*, 1913, **17**, 507
38. Magill, I.W. *Lancet*, 1926, **1**, 500
39. Flagg, P.J. *Arch. Otolaryngol.*, 1928, **8**, 716
40. Miller, R.A. *Anesthesiology*, 1941, **2**, 317
41. Macintosh, R.R. *Lancet*, 1932, **1**, 205; Boulton, T.B. 'Classical File', *Surv. Anesthesiol.*, 1983, **27**, 396; Jephcott, A. *Anaesthesia*, 1984, **39**, 474
42. Hill, W. *Br. Med. J.*, 1909, **2**, 1152
43. McIntyre, J.W.R. *Can. J. Anaesth.*, 1989, **36**, 94
44. Borland, L.M. and Casselbrant, M. *Anesth. Analg.*, 1990, **70**, 105
45. See also Mushin, W.W. *Anaesthesia*, 1989, **44**, 951–952
46. Rosenberg, P. *Berl. Klin. Wschr.*, 1895, **32**, 14
47. Magill, I.W. *Proc. Roy. Soc. Med.*, 1929, **22**, 83
48. Forrester, A.C. *Br. J. Anaesth.*, 1974, **46**, 413
49. Brain, A.I.J. *Br. J. Anaesth.*, 1983, **55**, 801; Brain, A.I.J. *et al. Anaesthesia*, 1985, **40**, 356

50. Chadwick, I.S. and Vohra, A. *Anaesthesia*, 1989, **44**, 261; Reynolds, F. *Anaesthesia*, 1989, **44**, 870; McClune, S. *et al. Anaesthesia*, 1990, **45**, 227
51. Werman, H.A. *et al. Am. J. Emerg. Med.*, 1987, **5**, 79
52. Tunstall, M.E. and Geddes, C. *Br. J. Anaesth.*, 1984, **56**, 659

10
Infusions and transfusions

Blood transfusion

The history of blood transfusion provides a good example of the inventiveness and vision of a few early pioneers, paving the way for many workers (often unnamed and unhonoured in their time), who subsequently made transfusion available to all.

Blood transfusions were first given to alter the patient's temperament! They were first described in animals (dogs) in 1666 by Richard Lower (1631–91)[1] and in man by Jean Baptiste Denis (c.1625–1704), Professor of Philosophy and Mathematics at Montpellier, France, and physician to Louis XIV in 1667, but using lamb's blood.[2] His first patient got better, but his second and third both died, and he abandoned the technique. The effects of incompatible blood transfusion in sheep is said to have been described in 1668.[3] The first successful transfusion for medical reasons was reported by J. Blundell (1790–1878), an obstetrician of St. Thomas's Hospital, London, in 1818.[4] Vein-to-vein transfusion was given by James Hobson Aveling (1828–92)[5] and by Higginson (of syringe fame) the following year. Autotransfusion, first described in 1874,[6] was often used in, for example, ruptured ectopics before World War II.[7]

A. Hustin (1882–1967) of Belgium in 1914,[8] Luis Agote of Buenos Aires[9] and R. Lewisohn[10] demonstrated the usefulness of sodium citrate as an anticoagulant for blood. They solved the agglutination problem which had prevented progress in transfusion. Apparatus for direct transfusion of blood was coated internally with paraffin wax to reduce coagulation, e.g. Kimpton's tube.[11] The anticoagulant heparin was discovered in 1916.[12] Glucose was first added to blood to prolong the life of the red cells also in 1916.[13] As with many other areas of medical history, the world wars provided a stimulus to thought and organization. The development of military transfusion by G. W. Crile in 1917 was a turning point in its involvement of anaesthetists in the total care of the patient. Prior to this they were largely concerned with sleep. After this they became increasingly involved in the prevention of shock, the maintenance of circulatory integrity, protection of organ function, pain control, and the other responsibilities borne today.[14]

In 1900, Karl Landsteiner (1868–1943)[15] of Vienna, later of New York, first observed agglutination of human red cells by serum belonging to other individuals, and described three ABO groups according to the two types of agglutinogens, their combination or their absence, which can cause agglutination when brought into contact with agglutinins in the serum. Landsteiner's intention was to provide haematological help in the diagnosis of diseases (for example, peptic ulcer was found more in patients of one blood group). The spin-off was safer transfusion. Landsteiner's realization of this was historically significant, eventually opening the door to organ transplantation. Landsteiner was a Nobel prizewinner in 1930. The fourth blood group (AB) was described by the Viennese physician A. V. Decastello in 1902[16] and confirmed by J. Jansky of Prague and by W. L. Moss of Baltimore in 1910.[17] The Rh system was discovered in 1939–40.[18] Signs of incompatible transfusion were highlighted in the early years of the twentieth century.[19]

Cadaver blood was used for transfusion in the USSR in the 1930s.[20] Not only was it ready available, but also it was free of fibrinogen and so would not coagulate. Blood banks were established in the 1930s in Moscow, at the Mayo Clinic in 1935,[21] by Bernard Fantus (1874–1940) in Cook County Hospital, Chicago,[22] and in 1939 in Barcelona during the Spanish Civil War.[23] Blood banks were set up in the 1940s in the UK, and the National Blood Transfusion Service incorporated into the National Health Service in 1948. Acid citrate dextrose allowed 21 days storage and was introduced in 1943.[24] Continuous drip transfusion was introduced in 1935.[25] The original glass bottles and rubber tubing gave way to disposable plastic sets in the late 1950s, which reduced the incidence of thrombophlebitis and infection. In 1946 there were about 200 000 donors in the UK, but today the figure is nearer 2 000 000.

As the twentieth century draws to a close, it is sad to record that modern transfusion services have been blighted in some parts of the world by the problem of cross-infection with the HIV and other viruses.

Intra-arterial transfusion was advocated in 1906 by Crile and Dolley and it was again advocated by Kemp in 1933.

Intramedullary infusion became a recommended alternative to the intravenous route in the 1990s, using the upper tibia or via the marrow of the manubrium sterni, especially suitable for shocked children. It has proved to be a method for transfusion of blood in the complete absence of a suitable vein.

For a full history of blood transfusion, see Keynes, G. *Br. J. Surg.*, 1943, **31**, 38; Maluf, N.S.R. *J. Hist. Med.*, 1954, **9**, 59; Diamond, L.K. *J.A.M.A.*, 1965, **193**, 40; Hutchin, P. *Surgery*, 1968, **64**, 685; Farr, A.D. *J. Roy. Soc. Med.*, 1981, **74**, 301; Marshall, M. and Bird, T. *Blood Replacement*, Arnold, London, 1983; Schneider, W.H. *Bull. Hist. Med.*, 1983, **57**, 545.

Blood substitutes

The first plasma substitute, gum acacia, was first used in 1919.[26] Polyvinyl pyrrolidone was developed by Helmut Weese and used successfully in the 1940s and 1950s but later discarded. The next major step in blood substitutes was stroma-free haemoglobin solutions; these still tended to have renal toxicity and it was not easy to obtain the correct position of the dissociation curve. Fluosol-DA, an inert emulsion of perfluorodecalin, and perfluorotripropylamine, was developed as a blood substitute which dissolved significant quantities of oxygen linearly with Po_2 according to Henry's law. It could unload its oxygen to tissues.[27]

Erythropoietin therapy (to avoid the need for transfusion) was described in the 1980s.[28]

Intravenous infusion

There has been steady development during the past 100 years, stimulated particularly by war experiences (e.g. Tom Shires' advocacy of fluid loading for injured soldiers during the Vietnam war). Saline was first used in the treatment of shock in 1891.[29] Hartmann's solution was a significant advance because it was more 'physiological', containing the same sodium, chloride, potassium and calcium content as plasma, with lactate to provide bicarbonate buffering.[30] The drip chamber was described in 1909.[31]

Haemolysis due to the intravenous assimilation of water (the original TURP syndrome) was described by C.D. Creevy in 1948.[32]

Hypodermoclysis (subcutaneous administration of saline) was used, when the intravenous route was not available, into the outer side of the thigh or retromammary tissue. It was facilitated by hyaluronidase. This was a 'spreading factor' which aided absorption of fluid injected into the subcutaneous and intramuscular tissues. It is a mucolytic enzyme which hydrolyses hyaluronic acid, an enzyme first isolated by Mayer and Palmer in 1934, but previously described by Duran Reynals in 1929. It is a testicular extract.

For the history of fluid administration during anaesthesia and surgery, see also Jenkins, M.T.P. In *Anaesthesia; Essays on its History,* edited by J. Rupreht *et al.,* Springer-Verlag, Berlin, 1985, p.102. For developments in infusion devices, see Rithalia, S.V.S. and Tinker, J. *Br. J. Hosp. Med.,* 1980, **5,** 69; Ballance, J.H. *Br. J. Hosp. Med.,* 1981, **26,** 411.

References

1. Lower, R. *Phil. Trans. R. Soc.,* 1666, **1,** 353; *ibid,* 1667, **2,** 557 (reprinted in 'Classical File', *Surv. Anesthesiol.,* 1976, **20,** 589.)
2. Denis, J.B. *Phil. Trans. R. Soc.,* 1667, **2,** 489
3. Flink, E.B. *Certain Aspects of Haemoglobinaemia,* Thesis of the Graduate School of Medicine of the University of Minnesota, 1945
4. Blundell, J. *Med. Chir. Trans.,* 1878, **9,** 56; Boulton T.B. 'Classical File'. *Surv. Anaesthesiol.,* 1986, **30,** 1000; Boulton, T.B. James Blundell and the introduction of the transfusion of human blood to man. 'Classical File', *Surv. Anesthesiol.,* 1986, **30,** 100–103
5. Aveling, J.H. *Trans. Obstet. Soc. Lond.,* 1864, **6,** 126
6. Highmore, W. *Lancet,* 1874, **2,** 89; Blundell, J. *Med. Chir. Trans.,* 1878, **9,** 56
7. Pathak, U.N. and Stewart, D.B. *Lancet,* 1970, **1,** 961
8. Hustin, A. *Bull. Soc. R. Sci. Méd. Brux.,* 1914, **72,** 104; Reinhold, H. and Bernard-Dichstein, C. *Proceedings 2nd World Congress on History of Anaesthesia.,* edited by R. S. Atkinson and T. B. Boulton, Royal Society of Medicine, London, 1989
9. Agote, L. *Ann. Int. Mod. Clin. Med. (B. Aires),* 1914–15, **1,** 24
10. Lewisohn, R. *Med. Rec.,* 1915, **87,** 141
11. Kimpton, A.R. and Brown J.H. *J.A.M.A.,* 1913, **61,** 117
12. McLean, J. *Am. J. Physiol.,* 1916, **41,** 250
13. Rous, P. and Turner, J.R. *J. Exp. Med.* 1916, **23,** 219
14. Boulton, T.B. *Proceedings of the History of Anaesthesia Society,* 1991, **9,** 54–58
15. Landsteiner, K. *Zbl. Bakt.,* 1900, **27,** 357; *Wien. Klin. Wochenschr.,* 1901, **14,** 1132
16. Decastello, A.V. and Sturli, A. *Munch. Med. Wochenschr.,* 1902, **49,** 1090
17. Boulton, T.B. *Surv. Anesthesiol.,* 1993, **37,** 122–130
18. Landsteiner, K. and Wiener, A.S. *Proc. Soc. Exp. Biol. N. Y.,* 1940, **43,** 223; Levene, P. and Stetson, R.E. *J.A.M.A.,* 1939, **113,** 126
19. Binder, L.S. *et al. Br. J. Anaesth.,* 1959, **31,** 217 (reprinted in 'Classical File', *Surv. Anesthesiol.,* 1975, **19,** 91)
20. Yudin, S.S. *J.A.M.A.,* 1936, **106,** 997
21. Lundy, J.S. *Clinical Anesthesia.,* Saunders, Philadelphia., 1941, p.606
22. Fantus, B. *J.A.M.A.* 1937, **109,** 128

23. Duran-Jorda, F. *Lancet*, 1939, **1**, 773
24. Loutit, J.F. and Mollinson, P.L. *Br. Med. J.*, 1943, **2**, 744
25. Marriott, H.L. and Kekwick, A. *Lancet*, 1935, **1**, 977
26. Bayliss, W.M. *Spec. Rep. Services Med. Comm., London*, 1919, no.25
27. Chilcote, R.T. and Gerson, J.I. *Anesth. Analg. (Cleve.)*, 1985, **64**, 4057; Jones, J.A. *Br. J. Anaesth.*, 1995, **74**, 697
28. Editorial. *Br. Med. J.*, 1990, **300**, 621–622
29. Lane, W.A. *Lancet*, 1891, **2**, 626; Horrocks, P. *Lancet*, 1893, **2**, 1569
30. Lee, J.A. *Anaesthesia*, 1981, **36**, 1115
31. Laurie, R.D. *Lancet*, 1909, **1**, 248
32. Creevy, C.D. *J. Urol.*, 1948, **59**, 1217–1232

11
Complications of anaesthesia and safety issues

It is to the immense credit of the speciality that complications in anaesthesia have been recognized, quantified and publicized, and that measures have been put in force to reduce them to an absolute minimum. Critical scrutiny of morbidity and mortality has been present from the beginnings of modern anaesthesia. The mortality surveys (such as CEPOD) and establishment of minimal monitoring standards (by, for example, Harvard Medical School and the Association of Anaesthetists of Great Britain and Ireland) are outstanding examples of this relentless search for safety at a time when surgery is performed on increasingly sick patients. This chapter catalogues just some of the milestones.

Notes on some complications of anaesthesia

Surgical emphysema during anaesthesia was first reported in 1912[1] during insufflation endotracheal anaesthesia. **Air embolism** was first reported in 1821 by Magendie,[2] and by Barlow in 1830.[3]

Vomiting was frequently described in early anaesthetic literature and was even occasionally fatal.[4] A classic paper on vomiting during anaesthesia was that by Morton and Wylie.[5] Fourteen years later, attention of practising anaesthetists was again drawn to vomiting and regurgitation as major contributors to deaths associated with anaesthesia.[6]

Peripheral nerve injuries were first recognized by Budinger[7] in 1894 as being due to malposition of the patient with consequent stretching and compression of nerves. The time course and predisposing factors were highlighted in the 1960s.[8]

Malignant hyperpyrexia was first elucidated by Denborough *et al.* in 1962.[9] Dantrolene treatment for this condition made a welcome appearance 20 years later.[10] Hyperpyrexia had been noted by Snow in his experiments with volatile agents,[11] and during ether anaesthesia in children in hot environments.

Accidental hypothermia was also noted in the early days, occurring during long operations, minimized by operating in a warm theatre and the use of a warming blanket. The critical theatre temperature to minimize a drop in patient temperature was later found to be about 21°C or 70°F.[12] See also Chapter 17.

Fires and explosions – for a concise history on this subject, see Macdonald, A.G. *Br. J. Anaesth.*, 1994, **72**, 710–722.

Hazards to medical and nursing staff began to be an issue in the 1970s[13] and led to the introduction of anaesthetic gas scavenging systems. There were a number of surveys suggesting that the anaesthetist and other theatre staff were exposed to hazards as a result of their occupation. They were thought to be more prone to coronary artery disease and suicide than their fellows in other occupations. Other hazards included liability to renal calculi, exposure to radiation, muscular and ligamentous strains as a result of lifting patients, the possibility of exposure to AIDS and hepatitis B antigen, and fatigue (which would result in a slow reaction time in an emergency and inability to form sound judgements). At that time, many individual anaesthetists worked excessively long hours. Chronic intermittent exposure to nitrous oxide was also known to interfere with vitamin B_{12} metabolism.[14] The evidence today that trace concentrations of anaesthetic gases and vapours continue to present a hazard to theatre personnel is controversial.

Development of safety issues in anaesthesia

Concerns about the safety of anaesthesia had been expressed since the first reported deaths under ether and chloroform in 1847 and 1848 respectively. An early book on anaesthesia by H. Lyman (Professor of Diseases of the Nervous System and the Theory and Practice of Medicine at Rusch Medical College, Chicago), entitled *Artificial Anaesthesia and Anaesthetics* (Chicago, 1881 and London, 1883) had a whole section on medicolegal issues. Dudley Buxton's book *Anaesthetics: Their Uses and Administration*, published by H. K. Lewis in 1888, also included a chapter on medicolegal aspects of anaesthesia.

In 1896 Frederick Hewitt[15] stressed the need for education as a means to help achieve safe anaesthesia. Although the need for anaesthesia to be included in the undergraduate medical curriculum was clear,[16] this was not adopted by the General Medical Council until 1912. Hewitt also persuaded the government of the need to ensure that anaesthetics should only be administered by qualified doctors, and a Bill was drafted to that effect. Its passage through parliament was prevented by the onset of World War I. In the second half of the twentieth century, an increasing public awareness and often unrealistic expectation of surgery without

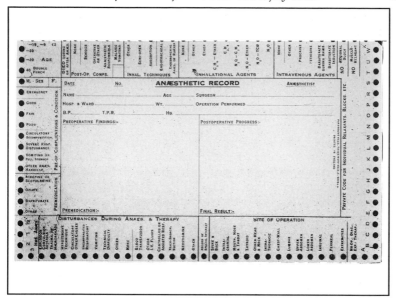

Figure 11.1 A Nosworthy card

morbidity and mortality led to increased litigation and a related interest in patient safety.

The International Committee on Prevention of Anesthesia Mortality and Morbidity,[17] and the Anesthesia Patient Safety Foundation[18] in the USA were started in the mid-1980s. The Australian Patient Safety Foundation first reported in 1988.[19] The International Task Force on Anaesthesia Safety has been active since 1990.[20] In the UK, the Association of Anaesthetists was influential in promoting the development of large-scale audit. The *Report of the Confidential Enquiry into Perioperative Deaths* (CEPOD) was published in 1987,[21] and several similar reports since that time. A crucial innovation in the 1987 enquiry was that both surgery and anaesthesia were audited together. It examined 4034 deaths that occurred up to 30 days postoperatively in three English regions over the course of a year. Some 500 000 operations were performed in this time. Only 3 deaths, or about 1 in 185 000 operations, were considered to be *solely* due to anaesthesia. The professional organizations in most countries have developed subcommittees to consider patient safety.

Anaesthetic records

Not surprisingly, these were seen from the beginning to be an important part of safety. John Snow's records of 1848–58 are a classic early example. Other pioneers in anaesthetic record-keeping included Harvey Cushing in 1895[22] and Ralph Waters in 1936.[23] E. I. McKesson's (1881–1935) 'Nargraf' machine of 1930 could produce a semi-automated record of inspired oxygen, tidal volume and inspiratory gas pressure.[24] Nosworthy's cards[25] (Figure 11.1) carried details of the patient, operation and anaesthesia, and had notches to allow rapid sorting with a knitting needle.

References

1. Woolsey, W.C. *New York State J. Med.*, 1912, **12**, 171
2. Magendie, F. *J. Physiol. Exp. Pathol.*, 1821, **1**, 276
3. Barlow, J. *J. Med. Chir. Trans.*, 1830, **16**, 19
4. Ellis, R.H. (ed.) *The Casebooks of Dr John Snow*, Wellcome Institute for the History of Medicine, 1995
5. Morton, H.J.V. and Wylie, W.D. *Anaesthesia*, 1951, **6**, 190
6. Edwards, G. *et al. Anaesthesia*, 1965, **11**, 194
7. Budinger, K. *Arch. Klin. Chir.*, 1894, **47**, 121
8. Britt, B.A. and Gordon, R.A. *Can. Anaesth. Soc. J.*, 1964, **11**, 514
9. Denborough, M.H. *et al. Br. J. Anaesth.*, 1962, **34**, 395
10. Lee, C. *et al. Anesthesiology*, 1981, **54**, 61
11. Ellis, R.H. (ed.) *On Narcotism by the Inhalation of Vapours*, RSM Services, London, 1991
12. Holdcroft, A. *Body Temperature Control*. Baillière Saunders, London, 1980
13. Cohen, E.N. *Anesthetic Exposure in the Workplace*, MTP Press, New York, 1980
14. Amess, J.A.L. *Lancet*, 1978, **2**, 339; Layzer, R.B. *Lancet*, 1978, **2**, 1227
15. Hewitt, F.W. *Practitioner*, 1896, **57**, 347
16. Buxton, D.W. *Br. Med. J.*, 1901, **i**, 1007
17. Cooper, J.B. *Can. J. Anaesth.*, 1988, **35**, 87
18. Cooper, J.B. and Pierce, E.C. *Anesth. Patient Safety Foundation Newslett.*, 1986, **1**, 1
19. Runciman, W.B. *Anaesth. Intensive Care* 1988, **16**, 114
20. Vickers, M.D. and Robins, D.S. *Eur. J. Anaesthesiol.*, 1993, **10**, suppl.7
21. Buck, N. *et al. Report of the Confidential Enquiry into Perioperative Deaths.* Nuffield Provincial Hospitals Trust and the King's Fund for Hospitals, 1987; Lunn, J.N. and Devlin, H.B. *Lancet*, 1987, **ii**, 1384; Morgan, M. *Anaesthesia*, 1988, **43**, 91

22. Beecher, H.K. *Surg. Gynecol. Obstet.*, 1940, **71**, 689; Hirsch, N.P. and Smith, G.B. *Anesth. Analg.*, 1986, **65**, 288–293
23. Waters, R.M. *J. Indiana St. Med. Assoc.*, 1936, **29**, 110
24. Westhorpe, R. *Anaesth. Intensive Care*, 1989, **17**, 250
25. Nosworthy, M. *Curr. Res. Anesth. Analg.*, 1945, **24**, 221; *St. Thomas's Hosp. Rep. (London)*, 1937, **2**, 54; *Anaesthesia*, 1963, **18**, 209

12
Cardiothoracic anaesthesia

Cardiothoracic anaesthesia has always posed special problems. The solution to these problems led first to benefits for all anaesthesia, and then to the early development of a subspeciality.

Thoracic anaesthesia

The problems of thoracic anaesthesia have been those presented by open pneumothorax, pulmonary collapse and secretions. The following are landmarks in their solution.

Open pneumothorax

Although there had been early attempts to operate within the thorax in an endeavour to remedy the effects of stab wounds of the heart,[1] progress could not take place until the problem of operating in the open chest had been solved. Some means had to be found to prevent the lung collapse that was inevitable with an open pneumothorax in a spontaneously breathing patient. It may come as a shock to modern anaesthetists to realize that the chest was opened in spontaneously breathing patients well into the 1950s, half a century after the development of the first ventilators. Anaesthetists of the first half of the twentieth century were slow generally to adopt such important technology into this area of practice.

The Fell–O'Dwyer apparatus for artificial respiration using a bellows and tracheal tube[2] had been used in thoracotomies in the late 1880s and 1890s by Rudolph Matas (1860–1957) of New Orleans[3] and by Theodore Tuffier (1857–1929) and Hallion of Paris.[4] Early attempts using insufflation methods also had some success. Matas modified the Fell–O'Dwyer apparatus by fitting a plug to occlude the glottic opening so that positive pressure could be exerted through the endotracheal tube, with a side tube for administration of the anaesthetic.[5] Tuffier and Hallion also demonstrated that intrathoracic surgery was possible using an insufflation method combined with a variable resistance to expiration, thus foreshadowing present-day methods.[4]

Ferdinand Sauerbruch[6] (1875–1951) (Figure 12.1), the pioneer thoracic surgeon of Breslau, assistant to von Mikulicz (1850–1905), experimented at the turn of the century on animals, using a negative differential pressure chamber which enabled surgical procedures to be carried out within the chamber while the head of the anaesthetized animal was outside. Lung collapse could thus be prevented. At the same time Brauer, in Marburg, experimented on animals by placing the head in a positive pressure chamber.[7] Sauerbruch used his negative pressure chamber to carry out surgery successfully on patients in 1904, the surgical team working inside the chamber, with the patient's head and the anaesthetist remaining outside. The chamber pressure was reduced by 7 mmHg.[8] Later he was to adopt the positive pressure apparatus designed by Tiegel,[9] which used the reverse method described by Brauer. The positive pressure method was developed further later in New York by Meyer[10] using a positive differential chamber to enclose the anaesthetist and the patient's head, allowing the surgeons to work unencumbered outside.

Franz Volhard (1872–1950) showed that this positive pressure technique usually caused hypercapnia. This led to the introduction of insufflation techniques by the neurosurgeon C. A. Elsberg (1871–1948),[11] who in 1910 adapted the animal work of the physiologists S. J. Meltzer (1851–1920) and Leopold Auer (1875–1948).[12] Elsberg also advocated direct vision intubation,[13] instead of blind oral intubation as practised by Franz Kuhn (1866–1929).[14] He also showed the need for periodic lung inflation during operation.

Mechanical ventilation

Apnoea had been produced by deep ether anaesthesia by Brat and Schmieden,[15] a problem which immediately called for some form of mechanical respiration. The use of controlled ventilation using a bellows and tracheal tube had been used in animals and in resuscitation in the nineteenth century. Janeway[16] carried out controlled ventilation first in dogs in 1909 and then in patients, but the method did not become accepted in anaesthetic practice until Guedel and Waters introduced a 'new intratracheal catheter' with an inflatable cuff in 1928,[17] after which Gale and Waters made the first report of one-lung anaesthesia for chest surgery in 1932[18] and Graham and Singer reported the successful removal of a lung during endotracheal anaesthesia in the following year.[19] Nosworthy[20] later promoted the use of controlled ventilation for thoracic surgery in Britain. Controlled respiration was possible using agents

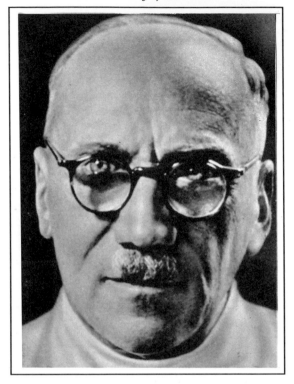

Figure 12.1   Ferdinand Sauerbruch (1875–1951)

such as ether[21] and cyclopropane with manual hyperventilation, but the introduction of muscle relaxants made it much easier. Automatic devices for rhythmic inflation of the lungs, or mechanical ventilators, were eventually used to overcome the need for manual methods.

Clarence Crafoord (1899–1984) of Stockholm reported his method of artificial respiration by means of Frenckner's mechanical spiropulsator,[22] developed in 1938 at the suggestion of the Swedish surgeon K. H. Giertz, who was a former assistant to Sauerbruch.[23] This was an early and successful ventilator. It was developed and simplified by Guedel,[24] Nosworthy[25] and Winston who advocated controlled breathing by intermittent pressure on the reservoir bag of a closed system, using deep anaesthesia with cyclopropane. This was a technique that had originally been introduced, using ether, by Guedel and Treweek.[26] Cyclopropane had great popularity during the decade following 1935 because, as a powerful respiratory depressant, it facilitated intermittent positive pressure ventilation. Other early ventilators were by Pinson,[27] Trier Morch (then of Denmark),[28] and Blease.[29] Muscle relaxants have now made controlled respiration straightforward, although they introduce complications of their own.

Bronchial secretions and one-lung anaesthesia

Gale and Waters first used one-lung anaesthesia in 1931 to isolate the lung undergoing surgery.[18] They moulded a standard tube in hot water to obtain a lateral curve and the tube was advanced towards the bronchus with the bevel towards the carina, stopping when resistance was met.

Advances in endobronchial methods were designed to prevent movement of infected secretions (often tuberculous) to healthy lung tissues, to allow their removal by suction, and to provide a quiescent lung for surgical access. A bronchus blocker was first described by Archibald, at the suggestion of Harold R. Griffith, in 1935.[30]

Modern use of endobronchial methods in thoracic surgery date from the introduction of the Carlens tube in 1949.[31] This flexible double-lumen catheter was used for bronchospirometry and was adapted for use in surgery by Bjork and Carlens.[32] Since then many other tubes have been described. They have been designed either to provide anaesthesia to the sound lung using endobronchial methods or to block access to the diseased lung using bronchial blockers.[33] Later development of double lumen tubes include those of Macintosh and Leatherdale,[34] Robertshaw,[35] Green and Gordon,[36] and Pallister.[37] Other approaches have included the use of a bronchial tampon inserted through a bronchoscope.[38]

Posture has also been advocated in the control of secretions, either to keep them in place as in the use of the sitting position in bronchiectasis of the lower lobes (often practised in children), or to encourage drainage towards the upper airways rather than to the healthy lung as in the prone position with head down tilt.[39]

Thoracoplasty was a widely employed procedure in the treatment of pulmonary tuberculosis with cavitation. The patient often had copious sputum containing the tubercle bacillus. Spread to healthy parts of the lungs was less likely if the cough reflex was present throughout operation. Ferdinand Sauerbruch is credited with the first paravertebral thoracoplasty for pulmonary tuberculosis. The operation had been first suggested by a German physician, L. Brauer (1865–1951). Morriston Davies performed the first such operation in the UK in 1912, and Tudor Edwards and J. E. H. Roberts the first pneumonectomy in the UK in 1935 at the Brompton Hospital.

Local analgesia was often used in cases where the thoracic cavity would not be opened, in the belief that the retention of the cough reflex would be beneficial. Paravertebral block was first described by Sellheim in 1906[40] and later modified by Läwen in 1912[41] and Adam in 1915,[42] although it was Kappis in 1912[43] who described what would be known today as true paravertebral block.

See also Mushin, W.W. and Rendell-Baker, L. *The Principles of Thoracic Anaesthesia, Past and Present,* Blackwell, Oxford, 1953; McLellan, I. In *Anaesthesia: Essays on its History* (edited by J. Rupreht *et al.*), Springer-Verlag, Berlin, 1985, p.126. For history of endobronchial anaesthesia, see White, G. M. J. *Br. J. Anaesth.,* 1960, **32,** 235; for history of the various tubes used in thoracic anaesthesia, see Pappin, J. C. *Anaesthesia* 1979, **34,** 57.

Bronchoscopy

A cylindrical metal tube, illuminated by candle-light to examine body cavities, was invented in 1807 by Bozzini (1773–1809).[44] In 1895 Gustav Killian (1860–1921) of Freiburg used a laryngoscope to peer below the cords,[45] but modern bronchoscopy was developed by Chevalier Jackson (1865–1958) in the USA and by Victor Negus (1887–1974) in the UK in the early years of this century.

Diffusion respiration was first described (in dogs) by Draper and Whitehead in 1944[46] and apnoeic oxygenation in man in 1947 by Draper[47] and later by Holmdahl.[48] The Sanders injector, using high-pressure oxygen and entraining air by the Venturi effect, was described in 1967.[49]

The fibreoptic bronchoscope was introduced in 1968 by Ikeda,[50] which has largely supplanted the older rigid tube methods, although the latter retain a place in the hands of thoracic surgeons.

Cardiac surgery[51]

Less than 30 years after the discovery of anaesthesia, surgeons turned their attention to the human heart. The first drainage of the pericardium for suppurative pericarditis was performed by Hilsman in 1875[52] and the first successful suture of a heart wound by Rehn (1849–1930) in 1896.[53] The first operation for relief of valvular disease was by Tuffier (1857–1929) in 1914.[54] The first pericardectomy for constrictive pericarditis was carried out by Delorme (1847–1929) in 1898[55] and later by Hallopeau (1876–1924) in 1921.

Survival of a case of mitral valve surgery was reported in Boston in 1923 by Elliott Cutler (1888–1947) and Levine.[56] Henry Souttar (1875–1964) carried out the first dilatation of the mitral valve in Britain in 1925,[57] the anaesthetic being administered by Mr Lindsay, a surgeon![58] But it was not until 1951 that surgery of the mitral valve became widely accepted treatment.[59]

Cardiac catheterization had been pioneered by Bleichröder in 1912 (on himself)[60], a feat of amazing bravery, especially considering that this was before antibiotics. Forssmann (1904–1979) continued this pioneering work in 1929[61] and Cournand established it in clinical practice from 1941.[62] Angiocardiography was started by Robb and Steinberg in 1938.[63]

The first ligation of a patent ductus was by Gross and Hubbard in 1939.[64] Surgical treatment of tetralogy of Fallot was initiated in 1945 by Blalock (1899–1964) and Taussig.[65] Harken removed a foreign body from the heart in 1946, and Clarence Crafoord (who also developed one of the earliest mechanical ventilators) surgically corrected coarctation of the aorta[66] in Stockholm. The first pulmonary valvulotomy for the relief of pulmonary stenosis was by Brock in 1948.[67] Valvuloplasty for mitral stenosis was performed by Harken and colleagues in the same year.[68]

Open heart surgery

Open heart surgery under direct vision with a dry field could only be undertaken when special measures were used to protect the brain from hypoxia during the procedure. Research into the value of generalized hypothermia was undertaken in the mid–1950s by Bigelow and colleagues in Toronto.[69] In Britain, hypothermia was used by Broom and Sellick[70] (see also Chapter 17). The other approach was to support the circulation either by the use of a cross-circulation from a parent,[71] which was only possible for the treatment of congenital abnormalities in children, or by the development of the artificial pump-oxygenator.[72]

Max von Frey (1852–1932) and Max Gruber (1853–1927) had developed an early animal heart-lung machine in 1885. The pump oxygenator was first used successfully in man in 1953 by John Gibbon (1903–73),[73] based on the Dale and Schuster animal oxygenator of 1928. Clarence Dennis had used a bypass in 1951 in which the patient died. This was a true turning point in the history of cardiac surgery. The technical difficulties were enormous, but were overcome by persistence, and improving technology with the development of new materials. The only other way of obtaining a still, open heart at surgery was deep hypothermia, to 20°C or below. This was used by Drew.[74]

In 1958 selective coronary angiography was reported by Sones,[75] and resection of an aortic aneurysm was pioneered by De Bakey in the same year.[76] Starr, using the newly developed pump oxygenator, or cardiopulmonary bypass, replaced the first aortic valve in 1963.[77] Saphenous vein bypass grafting began with Garrett in 1964,[78] but perhaps surprisingly, the internal mammary artery for renewing the blood supply to the myocardium was not used until 1970. The original pioneering work to enable the suturing of small blood vessels had been by Carrel (1873–1944) as far back as 1907.[79] The first cardiac transplants were carried out in man by Christiaan Barnard in 1967[80] and then turned into an almost routine procedure from that time by the intensive work of Shumway and colleagues.[81]

In the management of disorders of cardiac rhythm, the sternal pacemaker was used in 1954,[82] the first transvenous endocardial pacing in 1958,[83] and the first totally implanted system just a few years later.[84]

References

1. Hill, L.L. *Med. Rec.*, 1902, **62**, 846–848
2. Fell, G. *Buffalo Med. J.*, 1887, Nov., Section of General Medicine, Pan-American Congress, Washington, 1893 **1;** 237.; O'Dwyer J.P. *New York Med. J.*, 1885, **42,** 145
3. Matas, R. *Ann. Surg.*, 1899, **29,** 951
4. Tuffier, T. and Hallion, J. *Compt. Rend. Soc. de Biol.*, 1896, **48**, 951, 1086
5. See Mushin, W.W. and Rendell-Baker, L. *The Principles of Thoracic Anaesthesia Past and Present*, Blackwell, Oxford, 1953, pp.44–47; Matas, R. *J.A.M.A.*, 1900, **34**, 1371, 1468
6. Sauerbruch, F. *Das war mein Leben*, Kindler & Schiermeyer Gmbh, München, translated by G. Renier and A. Cliff, Andre Deutsch, London, 1953; Sauerbruch, E.F. *Mitt. Grenzgeb. Med. Chir.*, 1904, **13,** 399; *J.A.M.A.*, 1908, **51**, 808–815
7. Brauer, L. *Mitt. Grenzgeb. Med. Chir.*, 1904, **13**, 483
8. Sauerbruch F. *Zbl. Chir.*, 1904, **31,** 146
9. Tiegel, M. *Zbl. Chir.*, 1908, **22,** 369; *Zbl. Chir.*, 1908, **22,** 679; *Beit. zur Klin. Chir.*, 1909, **64**, 358
10. Meyer, W. *Ann. Surg.*, 1910, **52,** 34–57
11. Elsberg, C.A. *Ann. Surg.*, 1910, **52,** 23
12. Meltzer, S.J. and Auer, L. *J. Exp. Med.*, 1909, **11,** 622
13. Killian, G. *Münch. Med. Wochenschr.*, 1898, **45,** 844
14. Kuhn, F. *Dt. Z. Chir.*, 1905, **76,** 148
15. Brat, H. and Schmieden, V. *Münch. Med. Wochenschr.*, 1908, **55,** 2421
16. Janeway, H.H. and Green, N.W. *J.A.M.A.*, 1909, **53,** 1975–78; *Ann. Surg.*, 1910, **52,** 58; Janeway, H.H. *Ann Surg*, 1913, **58,** 927–933
17. Guedel, A.E. and Waters, R.M. *Anesth. Analg.*, 1928, **7, 238**

18. Gale, J.W. and Waters, R.M. *J. Thorac. Surg.*, 1932, **1**, 432
19. Graham, E.A. and Singer, J.J. *J.A.M.A.* 1933, **101**, 1371
20. Nosworthy, M. *Proc. Roy. Soc. Med.* 1941, **34**, 479
21. Guedel, A.E. and Treweek, D.N. *Curr. Res. Anesth. Analg.*, 1934, **13**, 263
22. Frenckner, P. *Acta Otolaryngol.*, 1934, suppl.20, p.100
23. Crafoord, C. *Acta Chir. Scand.*, 1938, suppl.54
24. Guedel, A.E. *Anesthesiology*, 1940, **1**, 13
25. Nosworthy, M.D. *Proc. Roy. Soc. Med.*, 1941, **34**, 479
26. Guedel, A.E. and Treweek, D.N. *Curr. Res. Anesth. Analg.*, 1934, **13**, 263
27. Pinson, K.B. and Bryce, A.G. *Br. J. Anaesth.*, 1944, **19**, 53
28. Morch, T. *Proc. Roy. Soc. Med.*, 1947, **40**, 603
29. Musgrove, A.H. *Anaesthesia*, 1952, **7**, 77
30. Archibald, E. *J. Thorac. Surg.*, 1935, **4**, 335
31. Carlens, E. *J. Thorac. Surg.*, 1949, **18**, 742
32. Bjork, V.O. and Carlens, E. *J. Thorac. Surg.*, 1950, **20**, 151; Bjork, V.O., Carlens, E. and Friberg, O. *Anesthesiology*, 1953, **14**, 60
33. Magill, I.W. *Proc. Roy. Soc. Med.*, 1935, **29**, 649; Rusby, L.N. and Thompson, V.C. *Postgrad. Med. J.*, 1943, **19**, 44
34. Macintosh, R.R. and Leatherdale, R.A.L. *Br. J. Anaesth.*, 1955, **27**, 556
35. Robertshaw, F.L. *Br. J. Anaesth.*, 1962, **34**, 576
36. Green, R. and Gordon, W. *Anaesthesia*, 1957, **12**, 86
37. Pallister, W.K. *Thorax*, 1959, **14**, 55
38. Crafoord, C. *Acta Chir. Scand.*, 1938, suppl. 54, p.65
39. Overholt, R.H. *et al. J. Thorac. Surg.*, 1946, **15**, 384; Parry Brown, A.I. *Proc. Roy. Soc. Med.*, 1948, **3**, 161
40. Sellheim, H. *Verh. Dtsch. Ges. Gynak.*, 1906, 176
41. Läwen, A. *Münch. Med. Wschr.*, 1912, **59**, 794
42. Adam, L. *Dtsch. Z. Chir.*, 1915, **133**, 1
43. Kappis, M. *Münch. Med. Wschr.* 1912, **59**, 794
44. Bozzini, P. *Der Lichleiter.*, Weimar, 1807
45. Killian, G. *Münch. Med. Wochenschr.*, 1898, **45**, 844
46. Draper, W.B. and Whitehead, R.W. *Anesthesiology*, 1944, **5**, 262, 524
47. Draper, W.B. et al. *Anesthesiology*, 1947, **8**, 524
48. Holmdahl, M.-H. *Acta Chir. Scand.*, 1956, suppl.212, p.1
49. Sanders, R.D. *Delaware St. Med. J.*, 1967, **39**, 170
50. Ikeda, S. *et al. Keio Med. J.*, 1968, **17**, 1
51. McKeown, K.K. *Can. Anaesth. Soc. J.*, 1982, **29**, 325; Mathews, E.T. *Curr. Anaesth. Crit. Care*, 1995, **6**, 186–191
52. Hilsman, F.A. *Schrift. Univ. Kiel*, 1875, **2**, 20
53. Rehn, L. *Zentbl. Chir.*, 1896, **23**, 1048
54. Tuffier, T. *Bull. Acad. Méd. Paris* (3rd ser.), 1914, **71**, 293
55. Delorme, E. *Gaz. d'Hopit.*, 1898, p.1150; Hallopeau, P. *Bull. Mém. Soc. Chir. Paris*, 1921, **47**, 1120
56. Cutler, E. and Levine, S.A. *Boston Med. Surg. J.*, 1923, **188**, 1023
57. Souttar, H.S. *Br. Med. J.*, 1925, **2**, 903
58. Ellis, R.H. *Anaesthesia*, 1975, **30**, 374–390

59. Keown, K.K., Grove, D.D. and Ruth, H.S. *J.A.M.A.*, 1951, **146,** 446–450
60. Bleichröder, F. *Berlin Klin. Wochenschr.*, 1912, **49,** 1503
61. Forssmann, W. *Klin. Wochenschr.*, 1929, **8,** 2085
62. Cournand, A. and Ranges, H.A. *Proc. Soc. Exp. Med. Biol.*, 1941, **46,** 462
63. Robb, G. and Steinberg, I.J. *J. Clin. Invest.*, 1938, **17,** 507
64. Gross, R.E. and Hubbard, J.P. *J.A.M.A.*, 1939, **112,** 729
65. Blalock, A. and Taussig, H.B. *J.A.M.A.*, 1945, **128,** 189
66. Crafoord, C. and Nylin, K.G. *J. Thorac. Surg.*, 1945, **14,** 347
67. Brock, R.C. *Br. Med. J.*, 1948, **1,** 1121
68. Harken, D.E. *et al. N. Engl. Med. J.*, 1948, **238,** 804
69. Bigelow, W.G., Mustard, W.T. and Evans, J.G. *J. Thorac. Surg.*, 1954, **28,** 463–480
70. Broom, B. and Sellick, B.A. *Lancet*, 1955, **2,** 452–455
71. Lillehei, C.W., Cohen, M., Warden, H.E. and Varco, R.L. *Surgery*, 1955, **38,** 11–29
72. De Wall, R.A., Warden, H.E., Read, R.C., Gott, V.L., Zeigler, N.R., Varco, R.L. and Lillehei, C.W. *Surg. Clin. North Am.*, 1956, **36,** 1025–1034
73. Miller, B.J. *et al. Med. Clin. North Am.*, 1953, **37,** 1609; Gibbon, J.H. *Minn. Med.*, 1954, **37,** 171; Kirklin, J.W. *et al. Ann. Surg.*, 1956, **144,** 2
74. Drew, C.E. *et al. Lancet*, 1959, **1,** 745
75. Sones, F.M. and Shirley, E.K. *Mod. Concepts Cardiovasc. Dis.*, 1962, **31,** 735
76. De Bakey, M.E. *et al. J. Thorac. Cardiovasc. Dis.*, 1958, **36,** 369
77. Starr, A. *et al. Circulation*, 1963, **27,** 779
78. Garrett, H.E. *et al. Cardiovasc. Cent. Bull.*, 1964, **3,** 15
79. Carrel, A. *Johns Hopkins Hosp. Bull.*, 1907, **18,** 18
80. Barnard, C.N. *S. Afr. Med. J.*, 1967, **41,** 1271
81. Shumway, N. and Lower, R.R. *Ann. N. Y. Acad. Sci.*, 1964, **120,** 773; see also Cooley, D. (1978) *Surg. Clin. North Am.*, 1978, **58,** 895
82. Zoll, P.M. *N. Engl. J. Med.*, 1954, **247,** 768; Weinrich, W.L. *et al. Surg. Forum*, 1957, **8,** 360
83. Forman, S. and Schwedel, J.B. *N. Engl. J. Med.*, 1959, **261,** 943
84. Chardick, W.M. *et al. J. Thorac. Cardiovasc. Surg.*, 1961, **42,** 816

13
Evolution of some subspecialities of anaesthesia

General surgery

The advent of anaesthesia opened the floodgates for surgical assault on sick patients during the second half of the nineteenth century. However, as always, relief from pain was purchased at a price and there was an actual increase in the number of perioperative deaths during that period, simply because of the increase in the number of operations performed. Widespread public and professional concern over safety during surgery led to a steady improvement in selection of patients and surgical techniques. The other, slightly later, great turning point of the history of medicine in the nineteenth century, antisepsis, eventually enabled the body cavities to be opened without certain death from infection (Figure 13.1). This in itself ushered in a new age of anaesthesia because it meant that more serious and prolonged operations were undertaken. From this sprang the need for muscle relaxation and intubation.

The abdomen was seldom opened before the 1880s. Billroth performed a partial gastrectomy in Vienna in 1881 and Reginald Fitz (1843–1913) described the surgical treatment of acute appendicitis in Boston in 1886. Dean sutured a perforated duodenal ulcer in 1894 at the London Hospital, and McBurney did an appendicectomy in New York in 1898. Conrad Ramstedt did the pyloromyotomy that bears his name in Münster in 1911 and Dragstedt performed a vagotomy in 1943 in Chicago.

Biliary tract surgery

This accounted for some of the earliest intra-abdominal surgery. The first successful cholecystectomy was by Lawson Tait (1845–99) in Birmingham in 1879[1] and this was repeated by Carl Johan August Langenbuch (1864–1901) of Berlin in 1882.[2] The first cholecystogram was by Evarts Ambrose Graham (1883–1957) of St. Louis in 1924.[3] The first exploration of the common duct for biliary calculi was by

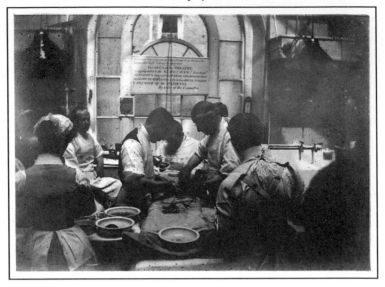

Figure 13.1   Nineteenth century operating theatre with bowls of phenol

J. Thornton in 1891.[4] The mortality of these operations was alarmingly high until the advent of antibiotics in World War II.

Day-stay surgery

This was extensively practised in Belfast and in Glasgow during the first decade of this century,[5] and also in the USA.[6] It has since developed into a mainstream of medicine in the closing years of the twentieth century. Although this is due in part to financial constraints, patients and their GPs recognize the advantages of avoiding staying in hospital if possible. Such surgery has been enabled by advances in surgical technique (e.g. minimally invasive, laparoscopic surgery), the advent of short-acting volatile and intravenous anaesthetics with minimal side-effects, and the increasing use of regional blocks for postoperative pain relief.

Dental surgery

Inhalational methods

In the early days anaesthesia was commonly used to facilitate the painless extraction of teeth. W. E. Clarke used ether for this purpose

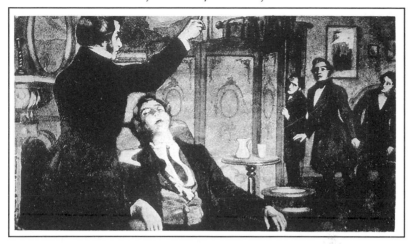

Figure 13.2   An early dental anaesthetic

in 1842. Horace Wells used nitrous oxide successfully in 12–15 cases prior to the disastrous demonstration in Boston in 1844 when he was hissed from the room as an imposter. From 1846 ether and later chloroform became the anaesthetic agents used in dental as in general surgical practice.

The first anaesthesia in England by James Robinson on 19 December 1846 was for the extraction of a tooth (see Chapter 2). In the following years anaesthesia for extractions was an important part of anaesthetic practice (Figure 13.2). The use of nasal inhalers for this purpose was developed by Coleman (1828–1902) and Clover in 1862.[7]

Revival of interest in nitrous oxide occurred as a result of the work of G. Q. Colton in the USA who formed the 'Colton Dental Association' in New York in the 1860s. By 1867 he had completed 24 000 cases without fatality when he travelled to France to attend the First International Congress of Medicine in Paris. T. W. Evans, an American dentist with a fashionable practice in Paris, learnt the method from him and in turn brought it to London, where he demonstrated it on 31 March 1868.[8] Colton's advice was 'Instruct the patient to take full deep and slow inspirations of the gas and hold the lips and nose so as to allow no particle of common air to enter and dilute the gas. By this means, anaesthesia will be reached in from forty-five to sixty seconds'. Both Alfred Coleman and Joseph Clover saw Evans at work. Clover began to use nitrous oxide in his practice, adapting his chloroform and air apparatus for the purpose.

Cylinders of nitrous oxide became available in 1868, when the firm of Barth compressed the gas and later when it was liquefied by Coxeters. Other pioneers of nitrous oxide anaesthesia include Edmund Andrews (1824–1904), who used it with oxygen to avoid the otherwise inevitable asphyxia, and Sir Frederick Hewitt. Hewitt advocated sound teaching and practice in the administration of anaesthesia, and in 1887 designed the first practical apparatus for giving oxgen and nitrous oxide mixtures.[9] E. I. McKesson (1881–1935) devised his demand-flow apparatus in 1926,[10] which was used up to modern times in some centres, while the British 'Walton' was an intermittent flow machine used widely in the UK.

The addition of oxygen to nitrous oxide in dental anaesthesia was popularized by Frederick Hewitt, and this is so much taken for granted today that it is difficult to believe that it was ever an issue! In the first half of the twentieth century, if pure nitrous oxide was administered the patient would pass through the stages of analgesia and excitement until the stage of surgical anaesthesia was reached. Oxygen was then added to prevent hypoxia, but the amount was carefully regulated because the margin between too light anaesthesia and dangerous hypoxia was known to be small. Some degree of hypoxia was accepted. This was no credit to that generation, since the physiologist W. S. Haldane had already stated in the early years of the century that 'hypoxia not only stops the engine, it wrecks the machinery' (i.e. causes organ damage in the brain, heart, etc.).

Intravenous techniques

Intravenous induction for dental anaesthesia became fashionable in some parts of London following the introduction of hexobarbitone, and later thiopentone. However, it was not until the introduction of halothane in 1956 or methohexitone in 1957 that outpatient dental anaesthesia[11] became modernized practice in the UK, with the benefits of adequate oxygenation and rapid recovery.

The dangers of fainting when the patient is held in the sitting position were widely emphasized by Bourne,[12] although Snow had described it on several occasions. (A faint in the dental chair was early shown to be a vasovagal syncope.[13]) This led to safer dental anaesthesia, because of the wide adoption of the horizontal position for dental procedures and the use of atropine to prevent such syncope. Knowledge of the physiology was the basis for the development of sound and safe anaesthetic practice.

Stanley Drummond-Jackson, a dental surgeon practising in London, used intravenous barbiturates when they became available.

Following the introduction of methohexitone in 1957, he developed the technique of 'ultra-light' sedation, the patient remaining in verbal contact with the adminisrator while dental procedures were carried out. Another approach was the use of 'relative analgesia' using subanaesthetic concentrations of nitrous oxide (less than 70%).

Diazepam began to be used for sedation during dental surgery between 1966 and 1968.[14] The shorter acting midazolam has been used more recently. The first local dental block[15] was given by R. J. Hall (Halsted's assistant in New York's Roosevelt Hospital) soon after the discovery of local analgesia in 1884. In Britain the first local dental block was given by W. A. Hunt of Yeovil.[16]

The speciality of dental anaesthesia

The Society for the Advancement of ˙Anaesthesia in Dentistry (SAAD) has been active since 1958.[17] The Association of Dental Anaesthesia (ADA) was founded in 1977. There is also a European Federation for the Advancement of Anaesthesia in Dentistry (EFAAD).

A number of committees have looked into the organization of dental anaesthesia. Those set up under the auspices of the Royal College of Surgeons of England include the Wylie Report (1978) and the Seward Report (1981). The Poswillo Report (1990)[18] was the result of a working party set up by the Department of Health. It made important recommendations concerning the training and accreditation of dental anaesthetists and of the standards of dental anaesthesia including use of monitoring equipment. The result of these efforts has been the gradual centralization of those surgeries equipped to provide full outpatient dental anaesthesia services.

For a history of faciomaxillary surgery and anaesthesia, see Ward, T. *Ann. Roy. Coll. Surg. Engl.*, 1975, **57**, 67.

Neurosurgery

The development of anaesthesia for neurosurgery, like that for cardiothoracic and many other branches of surgery, is a story of courage and determination by patients and doctors alike.

The first successful diagnosis and surgical removal of a cerebral tumour took place in 1885.[19] Sir Victor Horsley (1857–1917) of London removed an extradural spinal cord tumour for the first time in 1884. He began to develop neurosurgery as a separate speciality, having been appointed surgeon to the National Hospital for Nervous Diseases, Queen Square in 1886. This influenced the career and work of Harvey Cushing (1869–1939) of the Massachusetts General Hospital in Boston, who pioneered much of neurosurgery. Cushing introduced the silver clip to arrest haemorrhage in 1911 and pioneered the use of diathermy in 1928.[20] He also invented a pneumatic tourniquet to minimize bleeding from the scalp.[21] Walter M. Boothby was the anaesthetist for most of Harvey Cushing's surgery.

Walter Dandy (1886–1946) of Philadelphia described ventriculography in 1918[22] and air encephalography in 1919.[23] Myelography was performed, using Lipiodol, in 1922.[24] These are now seldom performed since the advent of computerized tomography and magnetic resonance imaging in 1973. Egas Moniz of Lisbon (who also introduced leucotomy) popularized cerebral angiography in 1927.[25]

The first planned operation for cerebral aneurysm was reported in 1932,[26] and the first localization of a cerebral tumour by electro-encephalography was in 1936[27] and then by radioisotopes in 1948.[28] Horsley preferred chloroform anaesthesia, whereas Cushing favoured ether. This was probably due to the current fashions in the UK and the USA respectively. A death under anaesthesia in 1893 stimulated Cushing to introduce the 'ether chart', a record of pulse, blood pressure and respiration during major surgery.[29]

Early pioneers of neurosurgical anaesthesia in the UK, many of them part-time general practitioners, included Zebulon Mennell (1876–1959), appointed to the National Hospital in 1911,[30] Maxwell Brown and John Gillies in Edinburgh, Noel Gillespie and John Challis at the London Hospital, Oliver Jones in Oxford, and Harry Brennan and Andrew Hunter in Manchester. Local analgesia was also used before the availability of muscle relaxants. Many considered them safer, as any respiratory depression caused by general anaesthesia would increase the intracranial pressure. Even the introduction of tracheal intubation in the 1930s and 1940s could not avoid hypercapnia from respiratory depression, and raised venous pressure due to expiratory resistance, again raising intracranial pressure and causing a swollen brain. The introduction of muscle relaxants and intermittent positive pressure ventilation transformed neuroanaesthesia and gave the anaesthetist almost complete control over the operative conditions enjoyed by the surgeon.

The concept of brainstem death was first described clinically in 1959.[31] It continues to provide occasional controversy and ethical problems for the anaesthetist.

See also Dott, N. *Proc. Roy. Soc. Med.*, 1971, **64**, 1051; Hunter, A. R. In *Anaesthesia: Essays on its History*, edited by J. Rupreht *et al.*, Springer-Verlag, Berlin, 1985, p.148.

Electroconvulsive therapy

Convulsions were first used in psychiatry in 1934 by Meduna of Budapest, who employed a relative overdose of cardiazol.[32] Cerletti and Bini induced fits electrically in 1938.[33] Bennett used curare in 1940[34], before it was used in anaesthesia, to modify cardiazol-induced convulsions. Holmberg and Thesleff first used suxamethonium for this purpose in 1951,[35] and it remains the standard drug today.

References

1. Lawson Tait, R. *Med. Times Gaz.*, 1879, **2**, 594
2. Langenbuch, C.J.A. *Berl. Klin. Wochenschr.*, 1882, **19**, 725
3. Graham, E. and Cole, W. *J.A.M.A.*, 1924, **82**, 613
4. Thornton, J. *Lancet*, 1891, **1**, 525
5. Calwell, H.G. *Br. Med. J.*, 1980, **1**, 115; Nicholl, J.H. *Br. Med. J.*, 1909, **2**, 753
6. Waters, R.M. *Am. J. Surg. (Anesth. Suppl.)*, 1919, **33**, 71
7. Clover, J.T. *Br. Med. J.*, 1868, **2**, 491; Coleman, A. *Br. J. Dent. Sci.*, 1868, **11**, 128
8. Evans, T.W. *Br. J. Dent. Sci.*, 1868, **11**, 196, 318; Colton, G.C. *Br. J. Dent. Sci.*, 1868, **11**, 256
9. Hewitt, F.W. *Anaesthetics and their Administration*, Griffin, London, 1893; *The Administration of Nitrous Oxide and Oxygen for Dental Operations*, Ash, London, 1897
10. McKesson, E.I. *Br. Med. J.*, 1926, **2**, 1113
11. See also Boulton, T.B. Outpatient dental anaesthesia from Clarke to Poswillo. *Proc. Ass. Dental Anesth.*, 1994, **12**, 38–61
12. Bourne, J.G. *Lancet*, 1957, **2**, 499
13. Lewis, T. *Br. Med. J.*, 1932, **1**, 873
14. Davidau, A. *Rev. Stomatol.*, 1966, **67**, 589; Brown, P.R.H., Main, D.M.G. and Lawson, J.I.M. *Br. Dent. J.*, 1968, **125**(2), 498
15. Hall, R.J. *New York Med. J.*, 1884, **40**, 643
16. Hunt, W.A. *J. Brit. Dent.Ass.*, 1886, **7**, 18–51
17. Sykes, P. (ed.) *Drummond-Jackson's Dental Sedation and Anaesthesia*, SAAD, London, 1979
18. Principal Recommendations of the (Poswillo) Report. *Br. Dent. J.*, 1991, **170**, 46–47
19. Bennett, A.H. and Godlee, R.J. *Med. Chirurg. Trans.*, 1885, **68**, 243
20. Cushing, H. *Surg. Gynecol. Obstet.*, 1928, **47**, 751
21. Cushing, H. *Med. News*, 1904, **84**, 577; Hirsh, N.P. and Smith, G.B. *Anesth. Analg.*, 1986, **65**, 288–293

22. Dandy, W. *Ann. Surg.*, 1918, **68**, 5
23. Dandy, W. *Ann. Surg.*, 1919, **70**, 397
24. Sicard, J.A. and Forestier, J. *J. Neurosurg.*, 1922, **20**, 721
25. Moniz, E. *Rev. Neurol.*, 1927, **2**, 72
26. Dott, N.M. (1897–1974) *Trans. Med.–Chir. Soc. Edinb.*, 1932, **NS47**, 219
27. Walter, W.G. *Lancet*, 1936, **2**, 305
28. Moore, G.E. *J. Neurosurg.*, 1948, **5**, 392
29. Cushing, H. *Boston Med. Surg. J.*, 1903, **148**, 250; Beecher, H.K. *Surg. Gynecol. Obstet.*, 1940, **71**, 689
30. Hunter, A.R. *Anaesthesia*, 1983, **38**, 1214
31. Mollaret, P. and Goulon, M. *Rev. Neurol.*, 1959, **101**, 3
32. Major, R.H. *History of Medicine*, Thomas, Springfield, Ill., 1954, p. 2
33. Cerletti, U. and Bini, L. *Boll. Atti Acad. Med.*, 1938, **64**, 136
34. Bennett, A.E. *J.A.M.A.*, 1940, **114**, 322
35. Holmberg, A.G. and Thesleff, S. *Nord. Med.*, 1951, **46**, 1567

14
Obstetric anaesthesia

Among non-pharmacological methods of analgesia, hypnosis has been used periodically since Anton Mesmer (1734–1815) first wrote about it in 1777, and childbirth without pain, employing relaxation and a naturalistic approach, is an old and frequently revived technique (Grantley Dick-Read, 1890–1959).[1]

The first Caesarean section, with a surviving mother, in England, took place in Lancashire by James Barlow, in 1793.

Sedatives and analgesics

Sedatives and analgesics were popular from the beginnings of anaesthesia, promoted by Simpson, and given to Queen Victoria (and countless others) by Snow. During the past century, chloral hydrate (introduced by Liebreich in 1869), tincture of opium and bromide formed a popular mixture, although designed to encourage sleep, rather than to relieve pain. This was to give place to barbiturates in the years following the introduction of barbitone by Emil Fischer and von Mering in 1903. Phenobarbitone appeared in 1912,[2] Somnifaine in 1924,[3] while Pernocton[4] and pentobarbitone came later.[5]

Morphine was used with success in labour[6] since its isolation by Seturner in 1806, and fetal respiratory depression was known to be its chief disadvantage. It was hoped, in vain, that papaveretum would be without this stigma.[7] Papaveretum was first used in obstetrics by Jaeger in 1910.[8] Morphine and hyoscine mixture was used in the technique of Dammerschlaf (twilight sleep) by von Steinbuchel of Graz[9] and by Carl Joseph Gauss of Freiburg, later of Würzburg,[10] following the use of the mixture as a complete anaesthetic.[11] Hyoscine alone was used in large doses in 1928,[12] but it produced far too much restlessness, due to central anticholinergic syndrome.[13] Pethidine was used by Benthin in Germany in 1940. Naloxone, a major advance in the treatment of respiratory depression in mothers and infants, was first used by Clark in 1971.[14]

The use of agents introduced into the rectum to relieve the pains of labour started, in France, in 1847[15] when ether was employed. Ether and oil had a vogue.[16] Bromethol was first used in 1927 and was closely followed by paraldehyde.[17] Ketamine was first used in obstetrics by Akamatsu in 1974.[18]

Various drugs of the phenothiazine group have also been used, and promazine was popular for a time. Synergistic prescriptions of drugs, such as rectal oil ether, morphine and magnesium sulphate, were at one time recommended. The use of diazepam in obstetrics was investigated by Bepko. Placental transfer of anaesthetic and analgesic drugs were not considered a problem to the fetus, although this attitude gradually changed as placental function became better understood in the last half of the nineteenth century.[19]

Inhalation methods

Inhalation methods (using stage 1 anaesthesia) were initially the prime method for obstetric analgesia. Ether was the first and was given by J. Y. Simpson on 19 January 1847[20] and by Dubois in Paris. Their example was quickly followed by others. Walter Channing, Professor of Obstetrics at Harvard, was an early advocate in the USA, and published his book *A Treatise on Etherisation in Childbirth*, illustrated by 581 cases, in the following year. After the introduction of chloroform[21] in November 1847, by Simpson,[22] the newer agent was used in childbirth in place of ether. It was felt to be safer and more pleasant for the patient. It certainly worked more quickly.

When Scottish Calvinists objected on moral[23] and scriptural grounds to the relief of pain in labour (*Genesis*, 3: 16: ' . . . in sorrow thou shalt bring forth children . . . '), Simpson quoted to them, knowing his Bible, *Genesis*, 2: 21: 'And the Lord God caused a deep sleep to fall upon Adam, and he slept: and He took one of his ribs, and closed up the flesh instead thereof.' Simpson thus yielded up the pride of place as the first anaesthetist in this area to God.[24]

In fact, the practice of administering some form of anaesthesia or analgesia soon became well established. For example, John Hobson Aveling (1828–92), a former pupil of Simpson, who later worked in Sheffield before moving to London, became a well-known figure in the history of obestrics and gynaecology with many publications. He was an early supporter of the use of chloroform.[25]

In 1850 discreet enquiries were made on behalf of Queen Victoria about the use of chloroform for the birth of Prince Arthur, and John Snow did administer the drug during the birth of Prince Leopold on 7 April 1853 and again at the birth of Princess Beatrice on 14 April

1857 (*Narcose à la reine*), a technique described in his book *On Chloroform and Other Anaesthetics*, published in 1858. On 20 October 1853 Snow also gave chloroform to the daughter of the Archbishop of Canterbury during her confinement. With the acceptance of anaesthesia by such eminent personages, religious objections to its use collapsed.[26]

The most common way of administering ether or chloroform in labour and childbirth was the open drop method, or by blowing air over chloroform vapour.[27] The drug was first used in the USA by A. K. Gardner in 1848. Divinyl ether was used by Wesley Bourne in 1935.[28] Cyclopropane had a short popularity in obstetrics just as it had in general surgery, especially in Montreal and Madison.[29] Trichloroethylene was found to be a useful analgesic in labour soon after its first use in surgery, and early reports came from Barnet[30] in the UK, and from London.[31] Methoxyflurane was been found to be safe when given in a low concentration for short periods.[32]

Nitrous oxide has had a long reign and of course is still a valuable analgesic today. First used in obstetrics in 1880,[33] its use was revived in 1915.[34] A method of self-administration was described in 1911 by that pioneer of anaesthesia, Guedel.[35] A significant advance was the introduction of the gas–air machine by R. J. Minnitt (1890–1974) of Liverpool[36] and its modifications. This method of self-administration held the field in the UK for some years but was given up because it could well cause fetal hypoxia. Nitrous oxide with oxygen was used in 1949[37] and the pre-mix of nitrous oxide and oxygen in equal volumes (Entonox) was advocated by Tunstall in 1961[38] and became extensively used.

Of the more modern non-pharmaceutical methods, the Leboyer technique called for calm, and soft music at delivery.[39] Underwater delivery has also proved useful for some mothers. A decompression suit was proposed in 1959 for relieving the pain of childbirth. Absolutely safe and pain-free childbirth remains a dream for the future. This long catalogue of worthy effort, extending back for more than 140 years, will surely be extended in the future.

Regional analgesic techniques

Regional techniques had an early vogue, to be eventually followed by an explosion of interest in the late twentieth century. Soon after Bier gave the first intradural spinal block in 1898, it was used in labour, and reported in 1900 by A. Kreis.[40] The so-called controlled spinal was used in 1928.[41] Saddle block was described in 1946.[42] Pudendal block was first described by Muller in 1908. Sacral extradural block was described for use in labour in 1909 by

Stoeckel,[43] paracervical block by Gellert[44] in 1926, and paravertebral block of T11 and T12 by Cleland[45] in 1933.

Eugen Bogdan (1899–1975) of Bucharest worked out the afferent pathways of labour pains[46] and gave continuous extradural sacral cinchocaine in 1931.[47] This work was independent of that of Cleland. Lumbar extradural analgesia was described in the USA in 1928,[48] and continuous caudal (sacral extradural) block again in the USA in 1938.[49] This was ably popularized by R. A. Hingson.[50] Continuous lumbar extradural block was reported by Flowers in 1949.[51]

Other milestones

Important milestones in the history of obstetric anaesthesia included the description of the *supine hypotensive syndrome*,[52] the description of the *acid aspiration syndrome*[53] and ways of reducing the effects of this by routine administration of an antacid mixture,[54] or H_2 antagonists[55] before anaesthesia.

Of the various obstetric manoeuvres, fetoscopy was first performed by Scrimgeour in 1973.[56] Amniocentesis was done as early as 1930.[57]

See also Heaton, C. E. *J. Hist. Med.*, 1946, **1**, 567; Poppers, P. J. The history and development of obstetric anaesthesia. In *Anaesthesia: Essays on its History*, edited by J. Rupreht *et al.* Springer-Verlag, Berlin, 1985.

Resuscitation of the newborn

John Snow used cold water to resuscitate a neonate in 1848 and used intermittent positive pressure ventilation with a catheter in 1849.[58] One of the earliest papers on such treatment was 'The asphyxia of the stillborn infant and its treatment', by Marshall Hall in 1856.[59] Intra-uterine respiration of the fetus, the rhythmical amniotic tide into and out of the air passages, was first demonstrated by J. F. Ahfelt (1843–1929), Leipzig obstetrician, in 1888 and then again by the Italian, Ferroni, in 1899.[60]

Virginia Apgar (1909–75) of New York City described her system of assessing the condition of the newborn baby in 1953.[61]

References

1. Dick-Read, G. *Childbirth without Fear*, 4th edn, Heinemann, London, 1976; Brown, F.J. *Antenatal and Postnatal Care*, Churchill, London, 1976

2. Loewe, S. *Dtsch. Med. Wochenschr.*, 1912, **38**, 947
3. Cleisz, L. *Presse Méd.*, 1924, **32**, 1001
4. Vogt, E. *Medsche Klin*, 1928, **24**, 24
5. O'Sullivan, J.V. and Craner, W.W. *Lancet*, 1932, **1**, 119: Irving, F.C. *et al.* *Surg. Gynecol. Obstet.*, 1934, **58**, 1
6. Kormann, E. *Monat. Gerburts. Frauenkrank.*, 1860, **32**, 114
7. Sahli, L. *Münch. Med. Wochenschr.*, 1909, **56**, 26
8. Jaeger, W. *Zentbl. Gynäk.*, 1910, no.46
9. von Steinbuchel, R. *Zentbl. Gynäk.*, 1902, no.48
10. Gauss, C.J. *Arch. Gynaek.*, 1906, **78**, 579; see also Greenwood, W.O. *Scopolamine-Morphine*, Froude, London, 1918
11. Korff, B. *Münch. Med. Wochenschr.*, 1901, **48**, 1169
12. van Hoosen, B. *Curr. Res. Anesth. Analg.*, 1928, **7**, 1963
13. Duvoisin, R. and Katz, R. *J.A.M.A.*, 1968, **206**, 1963
14. Clark, R.B. *J. Arkansas Med. Soc.*, 1971, **68**, 128
15. Pirogoff, N.I. *C. R. Hebd. Séanc. Acad. Sci. Paris*, 1847, **74**, 78, 79; Secher, O. *Anaesthesia*, 1986, **41**, 829
16. Gwathmey, J.T. *New York Med. J.*, 1913, **98**, 1101
17. Rosenfeld, H.H. and Davidoff, R.B. *Surg. Gynecol. Obstet.*, 1935, **60**, 235
18. Akamatsu, T.J. *et al. Anesth. Analg. (Cleve.)*, 1974, **53**, 284; Dundee, J.W. *Proc. Roy. Soc. Med.*, 1971, **64**, 1159
19. Caton, D. *Anesthesiology*, 1977, **46**, 132
20. Simpson, J.Y. *Mon. J. Med. Sci.* (Lond. and Edin.), 1846–47, **NS1**
21. Payne, J.P. *Br. J. Anaesth.*, 1981, **53**, 11S–15S
22. Simpson, J.Y. *Lond. Med. Gaz.*, 1847, **5**, 935
23. Farr, A.D. *Anaesthesia*, 1980, **35**, 896
24. Simpson, J.Y. *Answer to the religious objections advanced against employment of anaesthetic agents in midwifery and surgery,* Sutherland and Knox, Edinburgh, 1847; Caton, D. *Anesthesiology*, 1970, **33**, 102–109
25. Aveling, J.H. *An address to mothers, commending the use of chloroform; with refutations of some of the most popular objections,* 1853. Responsibility in administering chloroform. Correspondence, *Med. Times Gaz.*, 1857, **36**, 152; Chloroform in midwifery. Correspondence, *Med. Times Gaz.*, 1858, **38**, 671
26. Duncum, B.M. *The Development of Inhalation Anaesthesia: With Special Reference to the Years 1846–1900.* Oxford University Press, 1947; Atkinson, R.S. *James Simpson and Chloroform*, Priory Press, London, 1973
27. Little, D.M. *Surv. Anesthesiol.*, 1980, **24**, 272; Junker, F.E. *Med. Times Lond.*, 1869, **1**, 171
28. Bourne, W. *J.A.M.A.* 1935, **105**, 2047
29. Bourne, W. *Lancet*, 1934, **2**, 20; Griffith, H.R. *Curr. Res. Anesth. Analg.*, 1935, **14**, 253; Knight, R.T. *Curr. Res. Anesth. Analg.*, 1936, **15**, 63
30. Elam, J. *Lancet* 1943, **2**, 127
31. Freedman, A. *Lancet* 1943, **2**, 696
32. Major, V. *et al. Br. Med. J.*, 1966, **2**, 1554
33. Klikowitsch, H. *Arch. Gynaek.*, 1881, **17**, 81; Richards, W. *et al. Anaesthesia*, 1976, **31**, 933
34. Webster, J.C. *J.A.M.A.*, 1915, **24**, 812

35. Guedel, A.E. *Indianap. Med. J.*, 1911, **14**, 476; *New York Med. J.*, 1912, **95**, 387
36. Minnitt, R.J. *Proc. Roy. Soc. Med.*, 1934, **27**, 1313
37. Seward, E.H. *Proc. Roy. Soc. Med.*, 1949, **42**, 745
38. Tunstall, M.E. *Lancet* 1961, **2**, 964
39. Leboyer, F. *et al. New Engl. J. Med.*, 1980, **302**, 655; Editorial, *New Engl. J. Med.*, 1980, **302**, 685
40. Kreis, A. *Zentbl. Gynäk.*, 1900, 747; Doleris Malartie and Dupaigne, Report to Acad. Med. Paris, 22 January, 1901
41. Pitkin. G.P. and McCormack, F.C. *Surg. Gynecol. Obstet*, 1928, **47**, 713
42. Adriani, J. and Roma-Vega, D. *Am. J. Surg.*, 1946, **71**, 12
43. Stoeckel, D. *Zentbl. Gynäk.*, 1909, **33**, 3; Oldham, S.P. *Kenty. Med. J.*, 1923, **21**, 321
44. Gellert, P. *Monatschr. Geburtsh. Gynäk.*, 1926, **73**, 143
45. Cleland, J.G.P. *Surg. Gynecol. Obstet.*, 1933, **57**, 51
46. Bogdan, E. *C. R. Soc. Biol. (Paris)*, 1930, **105**, 25
47. Bogdan, E. *Bull. Soc. Obstet. Gynaecol (Paris)*, 1931, **20**, 35
48. Pickles, W. and Jones, S.S. *New Engl. J. Med.*, 1928, **199**, 988
49. Graffagnino, P. and Seyler, L.W. *Am. J. Obstet. Gynecol.*, 1938, **35**, 597
50. Hingson, R.A. and Southworth, J.L. *Am. J. Surg.*, 1942, **58**, 92; Edwards, W.B. and Hingson, R.A. *Am. J. Surg.*, 1942, **57**, 459 (reprinted in 'Classical File', *Surv. Anesthesiol.*, 1980, **24**, 275); Hingson, R.A. and Edwards, W.B. *Curr. Res. Anesth. Analg.*, 1942, **21**, 301
51. Flowers, C.E. *et al. Curr. Res. Anesth. Analg.*, 1949, **28**, 181
52. Hansen, R. *Klin. Wochenschr.*, 1942, **21**, 341; Holmes, F.J. *J. Obstet. Gynaecol. Br. Emp.*, 1958, **64**, 229
53. Mendelson, C.L. *Am. J. Obstet. Gynecol.*, 1946, **52**, 191 (reprinted in 'Classical File', *Surv. Anesthesiol.*, 1966, **10**, 599)
54. Taylor, G. and Pryse-Davies, J. *Lancet*, 1966, **1**, 288
55. Husemeyer, R.P. *et al. Anaesthesia*, 1978, **33**, 775
56. Scrimgeour, J.B. In *Antenatal Diagnosis of Genetic Diseases*, edited by A.E.H. Emery, Churchill Livingstone, Edinburgh, 1973
57. Menees, T.O. *et al. Am. J. Roentengenol.*, 1930, **24**, 353
58. Ellis R.H. (ed.) *The Casebooks of Dr John Snow*, Wellcome Institute for the History of Medicine, 1995, pp.22, 130, 152, 650, 702
59. Marshall Hall, (1790–1857) *Lancet* 1856, **2**, 601 (reprinted in 'Classical File', *Surv. Anesthesiol.*, 1977, **21**, 398)
60. Boddy, K. and Robinson, J.S. *Lancet*, 1971, **2**, 1231; Boddy, K. and Mantell, C.D. *Lancet*, 1972, **2**, 1219
61. Apgar, V. *Curr. Res. Anesth. Analg.*, 1953, **32**, 260 (reprinted in 'Classical File', *Surv. Anesthesiol.*, 1975, **19**, 401)

15
Regional techniques

Ether spray had been used by B. W. Richardson (1828–96) (Figure 15.1) in 1866[1] to 'freeze' the skin, and ethyl chloride spray for the same purpose in 1880 by Rothenstein, and in 1890 by P. Redard.[2] However, modern local analgesia began with the introduction of cocaine into medical practice in September 1884 by Carl Koller (1857–1944) (Figure 15.2), a 27–year-old trainee ophthalmologist in Vienna.[3] He was the first medical man to make use of and to publicize the analgesic properties of cocaine (which had been known for 25 years) to prevent the pain of a surgical operation, first using it for topical analgesia of the eye.

While training as an ophthalmologist, Koller soon began to share with his professor (Carl Ferdinand von Arlt) considerable dissatisfaction with the standard of the anaesthetists and of the conditions of anaesthesia they produced: restlessness during the operation and cough and vomiting afterwards. He began to realize that this problem would only be solved if he could find some drug which, when instilled into the conjunctival sac, would abolish pain. With this end in view he tried morphine and other sedative drugs, but of course without success. So the turbulent operating conditions under general anaesthesia continued.

In the summer of 1884, Sigmund Freud (1856–1939), a friend and contemporary who was working in a junior capacity in the neurology department of the hospital and who was later to achieve world fame as the originator of psychoanalysis, was busy investigating what was then a fairly new drug, cocaine, which had reached Europe from South America in the mid-1850s. It was an alkaloid extracted from the bush *Erythroxylon coca* which grew in Bolivia and Peru and was well known to the local Indians as a euphoriant and stimulant. Freud's studies led him to believe that it might be a remedy for morphine addiction as well as a tonic for his psychoneurotic patients. He wrote a monograph entitled *Ueber Coca* in August 1884. He knew that cocaine deadened mucous membranes but was not clear as to its effects on muscular contraction, and asked Koller

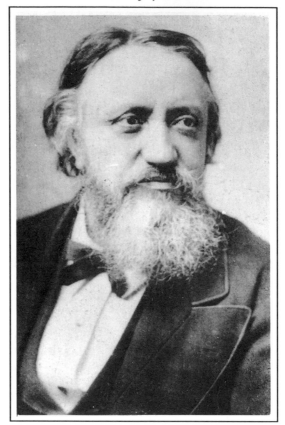

Figure 15.1   B. W. Richardson (1828–96)

to do some experiments to elucidate the problem. Freud then went on holiday while Koller set to work with cocaine.

He started by applying cocaine to his own tongue and was immediately struck, as others had been before him, by its strange power to deaden all sensation. In a flash he realized that this might be the agent he had been looking for to act as a local analgesic in his eye operations. He quickly set about investigating its analgesic effects in the experimental pathology laboratory on animals, then on himself, on his friends, and lastly on his patients. He satisfied himself that not only did it work but that it worked extremely well, and lost no time in making his discovery public. He wrote a short preliminary report[4] and asked his friend, Dr Josef Brettauer (1835–1905) from Trieste, to read it for him at the forthcoming

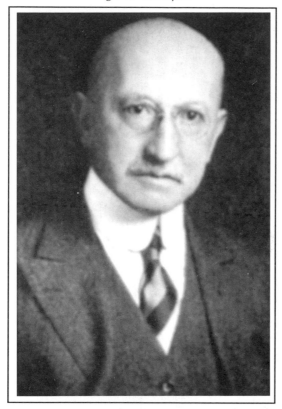

Figure 15.2   Carl Koller (1857–1944)[3]

Born in Schüttenhofen, then in Bohemia, a part of the Austro-Hungarian empire. Educated in Vienna, thought of studying the law, served for two years as a conscript in the Imperial Army and finally enrolled as a medical student in the University of Vienna. While still an undergraduate he published the results of some highly regarded experimental pathological investigations into the embryology of the mesoderm of the chick. Qualified as a doctor in 1882 at the age of 25 and became a member of the Department of Ophthalmology in the Allgemeine Krankenhaus whose director was Professor Carl Ferdinand von Arlt (1812 87).

News of his introduction of cocaine soon spread throughout Europe and the USA and Koller became a notable figure. But not notable enough for him to secure a senior post in the academic department of eye surgery to which he aspired and to which he was reasonably entitled. So he left Vienna and joined the Eye Clinic in Utrecht where he pursued his postgraduate studies under Professor Frans Cornelius Donders (1818–89) and his son-in-law, H. Snellen (1834–1908) and where he remained for two years. Koller was, however, a restless and somewhat awkward man and decided to try his luck once more in Vienna, but he found the going hard. His prospects were not enhanced by his involvement in a duel, fought with sabres, against a fellow reserve medical officer because of a personal quarrel. So, although Koller wounded his opponent and won the day, the illegality of duelling placed him in a difficult professional position and had an adverse effect on his advancement. Once again he decided to leave Vienna, this time for New York where he arrived in 1888 and where he spent the remainder of his active life. Soon built up a thriving hospital and private practice and established a solid reputation as a first-class ophthalmic surgeon. Took no further part in the development of local analgesia, leaving that to others. As time passed he achieved something of the fame his discovery as a young man rightly earned for him and he was awarded gold medals, scrolls and commendations from various academic bodies in Europe and America. Some controversy arose about this great discovery, but Carl Koller was its true begetter. Died aged 86.

---

meeting of the German Ophthalmological Society to be held in Heidelberg, which Koller himself was not able to attend. Brettauer's paper on 15 September 1884 caused a sensation and this was reinforced when, after a lecture, he gave a clinical demonstration of the use of 2% cocaine solution in the outpatient clinic. The following month Koller read two fuller papers before the Imperial Medical Society. Freud, whose interest in surgical anaesthesia was minimal, made no claim to the discovery.

Arthur E. Barker was using infiltration analgesia with beta-eucaine,[5] in 1899 at University College Hospital.[6] Reclus (1847–1914) in Paris[7] and Karl Ludwig Schleich (1859–1922) in Berlin (1892)[8] had popularized infiltration analgesia in the early 1890s, while nerve block had been employed by William Stewart Halsted (1852–1922) (Figure 15.3) and R. J. Hall in New York[12] the same year as Koller's pioneering work in 1884. The mandibular nerve was the first nerve that they blocked with cocaine. As a result of acting as their own guinea-pigs during their researches on the new drug, they became cocaine addicts. The problems with cocaine were its toxicity, clouding of the cornea, and (as was seen at this very early stage) addiction among those who prescribed the drug. Halsted extended the concept of nerve blockade, and was the first surgeon to use cocaine to block the nerves of the face, the brachial plexus, the internal pudendal and posterior tibial nerves. He showed that a reduction in the circulation of a part of the body, as by an Esmarch bandage, would prolong the effects of local analgesia. Halsted also demonstrated that for skin analgesia, intradermal injection ('the distension method') was superior to subcutaneous injection.

The first textbook on the subject was by J. L. Corning, and was entitled *Local Anaesthesia in General Medicine and Surgery* (Appleton, New York, 1886). H. Braun (1856–1917) introduced adrenaline in 1902 into local analgesia,[13] which was first isolated in pure form in 1897.[14] The term 'block' was first used in 1897 by G. W. Crile of Cleveland,[15] and 'regional anaesthesia' first used by Harvey Cushing (1869–1939) in 1901 to denote the production of analgesia by local anaesthetics.[16]

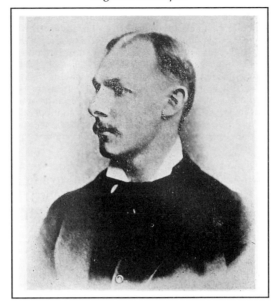

Figure 15.3 William Stewart Halsted (1852–1922)

Halsted's ancestors came from Britain in the seventeenth century and he was born on 23 September 1852 into a prosperous merchant family in New York City. Educated at Yale College where his athletic prowess surpassed his academic abilities. Deciding to study medicine, he entered the College of Physicians and Surgeons in New York in 1874 and graduated 3 years later. While a resident at Roosevelt Hospital, New York, in 1878 he became friendly with William H. Welch (1850–1934), later to become the first Professor of Pathology in the USA and the world-famous dean of American medicine. The next two years were spent in postgraduate studies in Austria and in Germany, where he visited the clinics of Theodore Billroth (1829–1924) and Anton Woefler (1850–1917) in Vienna, Ernst von Bergmann (1836–1907) in Wurzburg, Carl Thiersch (1822–95) in Leipzig, Richard von Volkmann (1830–89) in Halle and J. F. A. von Esmarch (1823–1908) in Kiel. When he returned home he entered surgical practice in New York City. Achieved considerable success and developed into a bold, extroverted and original surgeon. Was one of the first to recognize the importance of the discovery of cocaine and he and some of his colleagues commenced to experiment with the new drug on themselves, not realizing its grave addictive properties. In 1886, his uncontrolled addiction to cocaine led to his admission to a psychiatric hospital. Seems to have exchanged the craving for cocaine for the craving for morphine, possibly as a result of therapy, and remained a morphine addict off and on for the rest of his life.

On discharge from hospital his personality was seen to have changed and he now appeared as a slow, meticulous and rather morose man who gave great attention to the smallest detail of what occupied him. Found his way back to Welch's laboratory at the new Johns Hopkins Hospital in Baltimore in 1887 where he aspired to become Surgeon-in-Chief, but Sir William MacEwen (1847–1924) was offered the post (although he never took it up). Eventually in 1889 Halsted was appointed the first Professor of Surgery in the Johns Hopkins University and Chief Surgeon to the hospital. During the next 30 years of his life he made his clinic world famous and became one of the founding fathers of twentieth-century surgery, becoming mentor, guide, philosopher and friend to countless young colleagues, over fifty of whom eventually occupied chairs of surgery in American hospitals. His early enthusiasm for regional analgesia waned and in later life he always preferred to operate on unconscious patients. He died following a second operation for gallstones and obstructive jaundice.[9]

Among his contributions to surgery were his radical operation for the removal of the whole breast with its lymphatic drainage for the relief of breast cancer (1890).[10] In 1890 he introduced the use of rubber gloves into surgery, an idea borrowed from his colleague W. H. Welch, the pathologist (in an effort to prevent skin irritation from antiseptic solutions affecting the hands of his operating-room sister, who was later to become his wife).[11]

Local analgesics

Substitutes for the relatively toxic cocaine soon came. Oil of cloves (eugenol) was first used as a local analgesic in dentistry in 1890.[17] Giesel's tropococaine appeared in 1891, and Fourneau's stovaine in 1904.[18] Einhorn's novocaine (procaine) was described in 1899,[19] used in 1904, and popularized by Heinrich Braun (1862–1934)* in 1905.[20] Miescher and Uhlmann introduced nupercaine (cinchocaine) in 1929,[22] and amethocaine was described in 1931.[23] Lofgren and Lundqvist synthesized lignocaine in 1943, and Gordh was the first to use it in Stockholm in 1948.[24] Chlorprocaine appeared in 1952, mepivacaine in 1956, prilocaine (also first used by Gordh) in 1959, bupivacaine in 1963,[25] etidocaine in 1972, and ropivacaine in 1993.[26]

---

* **Heinrich Friedrich Wilhelm Braun (1862–1934)**

Has been called 'the father of local analgesia' and coined the term 'conduction anaesthesia'. Was born in Rawitch in Poland in 1862, and although intending to become a musician, he graduated in medicine in 1887 in Dresden, and after a period as assistant to Karl Thiersch (1822–95) in Leipzig and Richard von Volkmann (1830–89) in Halle, whose niece he married in 1888, became director of the Deaconess Hospital in Leipzig where his interest in local analgesia was developed, having been stimulated by Max Oberst (1849–1925) of Halle. In 1902 he introduced the use of adrenaline in local analgesic solutions of cocaine,[13] and in 1905 became the pioneer of the new drug procaine.[20] In this year also appeared the first edition of his classic textbook, *Local Anaesthesia*. The eighth edition was published in 1933. Preferred conduction (nerve) block to Schleich's infiltration. Appointed to direct the new hospital at Zwickau in 1906, and here he passed the remainder of his professional life. Introduced dental local analgesia into Germany. Described the anterior approach to the coeliac plexus (anterior splanchnic block) and was the inventor of the Braun splint. Also interested in general anaesthetics but realized their danger and devised an apparatus for the safe administration of chloroform and ether vapour.[21] President of the German Surgical Society in 1924 and retired in 1928. Died aged 72.

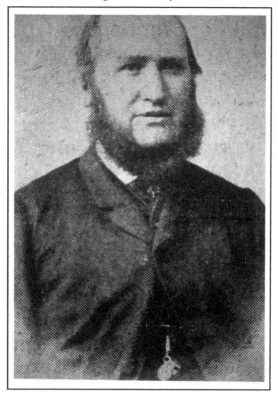

Figure 15.4   Alexander Wood (1817–84)

Techniques

Local analgesic drugs would have had very restricted use without the technology for their administration. Once again, a parallel development was provided which made regional blocks possible: the syringe and needle. The hypodermic trocar and cannula was described by Rynd (1801–61) of Meath Hospital and County Infirmary, Dublin in 1845,[27] and by Alexander Wood (1817–84) (Figure 15.4), a general practitioner of Edinburgh, who used a modified Ferguson syringe in 1855.[28] The latter also popularized hypodermic therapy for the treatment of neuralgia by injecting morphine near to the seat of the pain, a technique which was treated with condescending ridicule for a century until the discovery of peripheral opiate receptors. Luer all-glass syringes appeared in Paris about 1896; Luer-Lok syringes in the USA in 1925.[29]

Until the 1920s, it should be noted that regional analgesia was almost exclusively in the hands of surgeons. Anaesthetists were to develop various techniques for localizing the appropriate nerves for the block being performed. In the UK, R. R. Macintosh, J. Alfred Lee and R. J. Massey Dawkins were pioneers and practitioners of regional techniques. Prominent and pioneering workers in regional analgesia in the USA have included R. A. Hingson, J. S. Lundy, G. P. Pitkin, G. Labat, Lincoln Sise, J. J. Bonica, D. C. Moore, P. C. Lund, P. R. Bromage and Alon Winnie. The American Society of Regional Anesthesia was founded in 1920 by G. Labat and revived in 1976 with A. P. Winnie as president. The journal *Regional Anaesthesia* was first published in 1976.

For the early history of regional analgesia, see Matas, R. *Am. J. Surg.*, 1934, **189**, 362. For the history of limb blocks, see Bryce-Smith, R. In *Practical Regional Analgesia*, edited by J. A. Lee and R. Bryce-Smith, Excerpta Medica, Amsterdam, 1973, Ch.3. For the history of regional block in the USA, see Moore, D.C. In *Anaesthesia: Essays on its History*, edited by J. Rupreht *et al.*, Springer-Verlag, Berlin, 1985, p.128.

Spinal analgesia

Cerebrospinal fluid had been discovered by Domenico Cotugno (1736–1822) in 1764;[30] and its circulation described by F. Magendie in 1825, who gave it its name.[31] Although cocaine had been isolated from *Erythroxylon coca* in 1860 by Niemann and Lossen, and its analgesic properties described by Schroff in 1862 and von Anrep in 1880,[32] it was not introduced into medicine as a local analgesic until 1884 when Carl Koller used it for ophthalmology (see above). It was not long after this that it was applied to the nerves of the neuraxis.

The first spinal analgesia was by J. Leonard Corning (1855–1923), a New York neurologist, in 1885,[33] when he accidentally pierced the dura while experimenting with cocaine on the spinal nerves of a dog. Later he deliberately repeated the intradural injection in a patient, called it spinal anaesthesia and suggested it might be used in surgery: 'Be the destiny of this observation what it may, it has seemed to me, on the whole, worth recording.' This failed to influence his contemporaries. He wrote the first book on local analgesia, in 1886.[34]

Lumbar puncture was standardized as a straightforward clinical procedure by Heinrich Irenaeus Quincke (1842–1922) of Kiel[35] in Germany in 1891 and by W. Essex Wynter (1860–1945) in England in the same year.[36]

The first planned spinal analgesia for surgery in man was performed by August Bier (1861–1949)* on 16 August 1898, in Kiel when he courageously injected 3 ml of 0.5% cocaine solution into a 34-year-old labourer (Figure 15.5).[39] After using it on 6 patients, and to prove his faith in his method, he and his assistant Dr Hildebrandt each injected 2 ml of 1% cocaine into the other's theca, with courage bordering on heroism. Bier described his own post-spinal headache, attributing it to leakage of cerebrospinal fluid. They would have been worthy candidates for the Pask Medal! Bier advised spinal analgesia for operations on legs, but later gave it up owing to the toxicity of cocaine.

Tuffier (1857–1929)[40] and Sicard (1872–1929) in Paris soon afterwards extended its scope to include the external genitals and the abdomen. Frederick Dudley Tait (1862–1918) and Guido E. Caglieri (1871–1951)[41] of San Francisco, and also Rudolf Matas (1860–1957) of New Orleans,[42] were its first users in the USA in 1899, their works being published in the following year. Adrenaline was included to increase the duration and reduce toxicity of spinal analgesia in 1903.[43]

Stovaine (synthesized by E. Fourneau (1872–1949) in 1904)[44] (French, *fourneau* = stove), was used first in spinal analgesia in 1904 by Henri Chaput (1857–1904).[45] Novocaine (procaine), described by Einhorn (1856–1917) in Munich the following year,[46] was used in spinal analgesia soon after its discovery.[47]

---

* **August Karl Gustav Bier (1861–1949)**

Born in Helsen in Waldeck in Germany in 1861 and graduated in 1888 at Kiel where he later became assistant to the Professor of Surgery, von Esmarch. While there he supervised the transition from antiseptic to aseptic techniques in the operating theatres, following the teachings of von Bergmann (1836–1907) and Curt Schimmel-busch (1860–95) of Berlin. Became familiar with the work of a medical colleague at Kiel, Heinrich Irenaeus Quincke (1842–1922), who had established lumbar puncture as a safe investigation in routine neurological examination. In 1898 he gave the first deliberate spinal anaesthetic. Leaving Kiel, he became Professor of Surgery successively at Griefswald, Bonn, and as successor to Ernst von Bergmann at Berlin, and in the capital he was to spend the greater part of his professional life. In addition to his discovery of spinal analgesia, he invented the method of treating chronic inflammation by the method of passive hyperaemia with Esmarch's (1823–1908) bandage (1892)[37] and pioneered intravenous procaine analgesia (1908)[38] while holding the chair of surgery at Bonn. Was one of the great figures of German surgery, as teacher, lecturer and operator (Hon. FRCS (Eng.), 1913). Introduced the 'tin helmet' into the German Army in World War I. In later life he came to hold unorthodox ideas, advocated physical education, callisthenics, etc. and deviated from the views of his colleagues. Died, aged 88, at Sauer in the German Democratic Republic.

Aus der Königlichen chirurgischen Klinik zu Kiel.

Versuche über Cocainisirung des Rückenmarkes.

Von

Prof. Dr. August Bier.

Die Schleich'sche Infiltrations- und die Oberst'sch regionäre Cocainanästhesie haben die gefährliche allgemeine Na kose in sehr wesentlicher und erfreulicher Weise beschränkt. Abe für „grosse" Operationen sind beide Verfahren doch nur im geringe Grade verwendbar. Ich habe den Versuch gemacht, durch Cocaini sirung des Rückenmarkes grosse Strecken des Körpers unempfind lich gegen Schmerz zu machen. Dies wurde in folgender Weis ausgeführt:

Bei dem in Seitenlage befindlichen Kranken wird die Quincke sche Lumbalpunktion in bekannter Weise vorgenommen. Di Hohlnadel wählt man sehr dünn. Nachdem sie in den Sac der Rückenmarkshäute eingedrungen ist, entfernt man den Stöpse welcher die Lichtung der Nadel verschliesst, und setzt sofort de Finger auf die Mündung, damit möglichst wenig Liquor cerebr spinalis ausfliesst. Mit einer Pravaz'schen Spritze, welche gena auf die Punktionsnadel passt, wird die gewünschte Menge Cocai eingespritzt. Dabei muss man natürlich bei der Länge der Nad so viel Cocainlösung mehr nehmen, als die Lichtung derselben fass (Bei unserer Nadel 1½ Theilstriche der Pravaz'schen Spritz Damit das Cocain nicht aus dem Stichkanale der Rückenmarkshäu in die Gewebe sickert, lässt man die Nadel mit der daraufsitzend Spritze 2 Minuten stecken und entfernt sie dann. Die Stichöffnun in der Haut wird mit Collodium verklebt.

Die Lumbalpunktion wird unter Schleich's Infiltrationsa ästhesie schmerzlos ausgeführt. Zuerst wird die Haut, dann werd mit einer langen Nadel die übrigen Weichtheile bis auf die Wirb säule infiltrirt.

Fig. 2. August Bier's first paper on true spinal anesthesia, first page (from Deutsche Zts f. Chir., 51:361-369 [Apr.] 1899).

Bullard, O. K.: Intravenous Anesthesia in Office Practice. *Anes and Analg.*, 19:26-30 (Jan.-Feb.) 1940.

[Clarck, Timothy]: A letter, written to the publisher by the learn and experienced Dr. Timothy Clarck, one of His Majesty's physicians ordinary, concerning some anatomical inventions and observations, p

101

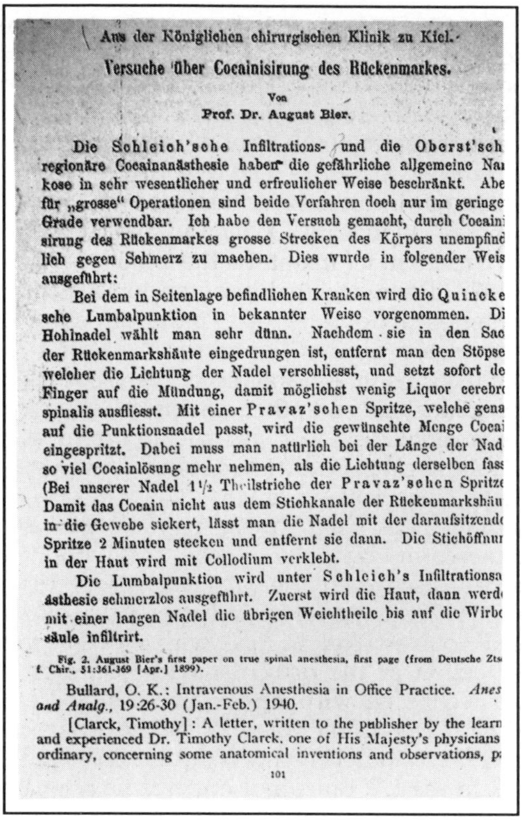

Figure 15.5 Reproduction of Bier's classic paper

Alfred E. Barker (1850–1916), of London, the leading pioneer of spinal analgesia in Britain, was the first to realize (in 1906–7) the importance of the curves of the vertebral canal and the use of gravity in control of level of analgesia.[48] He introduced 'heavy' Stovaine solutions in 1907 in Britain. Other early users of spinal analgesia in the UK were Robert Jones, a Liverpool orthopaedic surgeon,[49] H. P. Dean, of the London Hospital[50] and Tyrrell Gray in children.[51] Babcock of Philadelphia was the first to use light solutions, his formula containing Stovaine, alcohol, lactic acid, strychnine, etc.[52]

Apart from the experimental work of these pioneers, spinal analgesia was little used until the work of Gaston Labat

(1877–1934)* in 1921.[54] He urged the use of novocaine (procaine) crystals dissolved in cerebrospinal fluid, together with barbotage and early move into the Trendelenburg position. George Pitkin, a pupil of Babcock, developed his light (spinocaine) and heavy (duracaine) solutions, and the use of the fine-bore, short-bevel needle (1927).[55]

Chen and Schmidt introduced ephedrine in 1923,[56] and as spinal anaesthesia gained popularity, Ocherblad and Dillon[57] and Rudolf and Graham[58] used it to maintain the blood pressure in spinal analgesia in 1927. The associated hypotension was first thought to be due to anterior abdominal wall paralysis causing decreased intrathoracic pressure during inspiration.[59] Later it was correctly suggested that the cause was paralysis of the vasoconstrictor nerves supplying the splanchnic and other vessels.[60] Gaston Labat insisted that the hypotension itself was not so important as the cerebral ischaemia it might cause, and introduced a head-down tilt – a characteristically safe manoeuvre.

Spinal analgesia was used for surgery of the head, neck and thorax by Jonnesco in 1909[61] and Koster, the Brooklyn surgeon, in 1928.[62] Miescher discovered the analgesic properties of Percaine (nupercaine) in 1929. It was used in hyperbaric solution by Keyes and McLelland[63] of New York in 1930, with great success, partly due to the longer action of the drug. Howard Jones of London also published his technique with nupercaine, using hypobaric solutions, in 1930.[64] Nupercaine was also taken up by Kirschner of Heidelberg in 1932,[65] and Sebrechts of Bruges in 1934.[66] Etherington Wilson's work in the UK on spinal nupercaine appeared in 1934.[67] Walter Lemmon's first account of continuous spinal analgesia (using novocaine) was published in 1940,[68] although Dean, of the London Hospital, had described this technique as early as 1907.[69]

---

* **Gaston Labat (1877–1934)**

Born in the Seychelles and graduated at Montpellier. Took up the study of medicine at the age of 37 in 1914 after running a successful pharmacy in Mauritius. Became anaesthetist to Victor Pauchet (1869–1936), surgeon to the St. Michael Hospital in Paris, and was co-author with Pauchet of the later editions of the latter's book, *L'Anaesthésie Régionale* (Doin, Paris, 1921).[53] Was invited to the Mayo Clinic in 1920 and became Special Lecturer on Regional Anaesthesia there. Wrote his classic book *Regional Anesthesia; Its Technique and Clinical Application* in 1922. Subsequently became Clinical Professor of Surgery (Anesthesia) at New York University and worked at the Bellevue Hospital. Founded American Society of Regional Anesthesia in 1923. Died in October 1934 in New York. A third (posthumous) edition of his book was published in 1967, edited by J. Adriani, and a fourth in 1985. His book, outstanding in its time, had a great influence on the development and acceptance of regional analgesia. In 1922 its main readers were surgeons. Only in later years was regional analgesia practised by anaesthetists.

Lincoln Fleetwood Sise (1874–1942) of Boston popularized ame-thocaine (tetracaine),[70] which was synthesized by Eisleb in 1928.[71] Bupivacaine was first used for intradural block in 1966.[72]

In the UK, intradural spinal analgesia was for many years under a cloud, partly because of the tendency to litigation should compli-cations follow. An example was the Woolley and Roe case in the early 1950s in which paraplegia followed spinal analgesia in two patients operated upon on the same day, and was thought at the time to be due to contamination of the analgesic solution by phenol which had entered the ampoules through minute cracks in the glass.[73]

The articles 'The grave spinal cord paralyses caused by spinal analgesia' by Foster Kennedy[74] and 'Neurological complications after spinal anaesthesia'[75] also had an important effect on the climate of opinion. They stimulated Dripps (1911–74) and Vandam[76] to write in 1954 their article entitled 'The long-term follow-up of patients who received 10,098 spinal analgesics: failure to discover major neurological sequelae'. A later reassessment of the Woolley and Roe case[77] showed that it was unlikely that phenol was the cause of postoperative paralysis. Therapeutic injection of phenol for chronic pain does not give rise to the same clinical picture. A much more likely explanation is that the apparatus used was sterilized by boiling in a sterilizer which had been contaminated with acid substances used to prevent scale formation.

Epidural (extradural) analgesia

Sacral block

Fernand Cathelin (1873–1945),[78] a urological surgeon, and Jean-Athanese Sicard (1872–1929),[79] a neurologist, both working inde-pendently in Paris in 1901, were the first to use the sacral approach to the epidural space. This was some years before the lumbar route came into use. Sacral block was then employed in Germany by Stoekel[80] in 1909 and Läwen[81] in 1910, before it was popularized by Gaston Labat in his book[82] of 1923. The use of the technique in infants was described by Campbell in 1933.[83] The method of continuous caudal analgesia was developed by Hingson in 1943.[84]

Lumbar epidural block

It will never be known for certain whether Corning deposited cocaine into the intradural or extradural space in 1885.[33] Heile[85] suggested an approach to the extradural space through the inter-vertebral foramen, but the credit for its clinical use is due to Fidel Pagés,[86] of Madrid in 1921. On his death on active service soon after

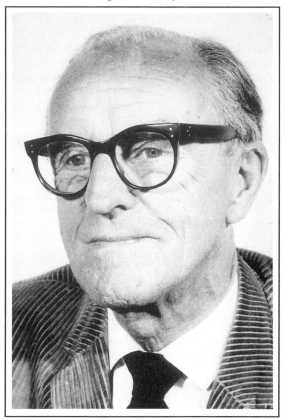

Figure 15.6   J. Alfred Lee (1906–89)

Born near Liverpool, son of a Congregational minister. Qualified from Newcastle upon Tyne medical school (University of Durham) in 1927. As a general practitioner in Southend-on-Sea during the 1930s, he maintained his interest in anaesthesia, and in 1939 became a whole-time specialist in the Emergency Medical Service on the east coast of England during hostilities. When he asked the Hospital Board for a syringe with which to inject thiopentone, he was told that there were no funds for these new and unnecessary techniques! (He then purchased his own syringe and used it throughout the war years.) Received the same response when he asked for a laryngoscope! During this time he wrote the first edition of the *Synopsis of Anaesthesia*, with the far-sighted intention of helping anaesthetists who were returning to civilian life from World War II. John Wright and Sons Ltd of Bristol published the *Synopsis of Anaesthesia*. It not only achieved its aim, but became the main encyclopaedic reference work in English (and many other languages) on the subject of anaesthesia. A superb teacher, and through the *Synopsis* was subsequently able to teach safe anaesthesia to scores of thousands of anaesthetists throughout the world.

Appointed consultant anaesthetist to the new British National Health Service in 1948, in Southend Hospital, a post he held with distinction until retirement in 1971.

Assistant Editor and later Chairman of the Editorial Board of *Anaesthesia*, a member of the Board and Examiner for the Fellowship of the Faculty of Anaesthetists, President of the Association of Anaesthetists of Great Britain and Ireland, and President of the History of Anaesthesia Society. Opened the first theatre post-operative observation ward in Europe in 1956[95] and an early pre-anaesthetic outpatient clinic.[96] A powerful advocate of extradural analgesia, with particular reference to safety precautions in this technique. What was remarkable about him was that he was an enthusiastic and expert teacher in the decades when teaching was shunned by those practising anaesthesia for fear that their pupils would steal their private practice.

---

publication of his paper, the innovation was forgotten until the work of the Italian surgeon, Achille Mario Dogliotti[87] in Turin, and that of Aburel[88] in Roumania in 1931. The technique then became widespread due to the work of, among others, Odom[89] in the USA and Massey Dawkins[90] in Britain. Influential textbooks were published by Moore, D.C. *Regional Block*, Thomas, Springfield, Ill., 1953; Bromage, P.R. *Spinal Epidural Analgesia*, Livingstone, Edinburgh, 1954; Bonica, J.J. *Clinical Applications of Diagnostic and Therapeutic Nerve Blocks*, Thomas, Springfield, Ill., 1959; and Lund, P.C. *Peridural Anesthesia and Analgesia*, Thomas, Springfield, Ill., 1966.

Curbelo[91] of Cuba was the first to insert a ureteric catheter into the epidural space to allow continuous block, using the Tuohy needle[92] first designed for intrathecal use, adapted to allow the use of smaller bore catheters.[93] The first report of the injection of opiates into the epidural space came from Jerusalem[94] in 1979.

For a history of spinal and epidural analgesia, see the book by J. Alfred Lee (1906–89) (Figure 15.6) and his co-authors Atkinson, R. S. and Watt, M. J. *Sir Robert Macintosh's Lumbar Puncture and Spinal Analgesia, Intradural and Extradural*, 5th edn, Churchill Livingstone, Edinburgh, 1985, Ch. 1.

Intravenous regional analgesia

First described by Bier in 1908[38] using procaine, though it never became widely used. Recent popularity follows the introduction of lignocaine, when Riha[97] in 1962 and Holmes[98] in 1963 showed that the new drug produced a more reliable analgesia. Prilocaine has become the agent of choice,[99] but bupivacaine is not recommended owing to its potential toxicity.[100]

References

1. Richardson B.W. *Med. Times. Gaz.*, 1866, **1**, 115
2. Redard, P. Vera *Xth. Int. Med. Cong.*, 1890, **5**, 14, abstract 71
3. See also Koller, C. *J.A.M.A.*, 1928, **90**, 1742; *J.A.M.A.* 1941, **117**, 1284; Koller-Becker, H. *Psychoanal. Q.*, 1963, **32**, 509; Liljestrand, G. *Acta*

Physiol. Scand., 1967, suppl. 299, **3**, 30; Wyklicky, H. and Skopec, M. In *Regional Anaesthesia, 1884–1984*, edited by D. B. Scott *et al.*, Production ICM AB, Sodertalje, 1984; McAuley, J.F. *Br. Dent. J.*, 1985, **158**, 339

4. Koller, C. *Klin. Mbl. Augen.*, 1884, **22**, 60; *Wien. Med. Wochenschr.*, 1884, **34**, 1276, 1309 (translated and reprinted in 'Classical File', *Surv. Anesthesiol.*, 1963, **7**, 74 and *ibid.* 1965, **9**, 287); *Lancet*, 1884, **2**, 990; Boulton, T.B. 'Classical File', *Surv. Anesthesiol.*, 1984, **28**, 346–354

5. Vinci, G. *Berlin Klin. Wochenschr.*, 1896, **27**, 84

6. Barker, A.E. *Lancet*, 1899, **1**, 282

7. Reclus, P. *Gaz. Hebd. Med. (Paris)*, 1890, p.106; *La Cocaine en Chirurgie*, Masson, Paris, 1895

8. Schleich, K.L. *Verh. Dtsch. Ges. Chir.*, 1892, **21**, 121; *Gesellsch. f. Chir.*, 1892, **21**, 121; *Therap. Monats.*, 1894, **8**, 429; *Schmerzlöse Operationen*, Springer, Berlin, 1894

9. Glen, F. and Dillon, L.D. *Surg. Gynecol. Obstet.*, 1980, **151**, 518

10. Halsted, W.S. *Johns Hopkins Hosp. Rep.*, 1890, **2**, 255

11. See also MacCallum, W.G. *William Stewart Halsted*, The Johns Hopkins Press, Baltimore, 1930; Boise, M. Halsted as an anesthetist knew him, *Surgery*, 1952, **32**, 498; Halsted Centenary Meeting, *Proc. Roy. Soc. Med.*, 1952, **45**, 555; Olch, P.D. *Anesthesiology*, 1975, **42**, 479; letter from W. S. Halsted to Sir William Osler in Fulton, J. *Harvey Cushing: A Biography.* Blackwell, Oxford, 1946, p.142; Hirsch, N.P. and Smith, G.B. *Anesth. Analg.*, 1986, **65**, 288–93; William Stewart Halsted and the Germanic influence on training and education programs in surgery, *Surg. Gynecol. Obstet.*, 1978, **147**, 602; *Bull. N. Y. Acad. Med.*, 1984, **60**, 176; Matas, R. *Am. J. Surg.*, 1934, **25**, 195, 362; Matas, R. *Bull. Johns Hopkins Hosp.*, 1925, **36**, 1; Matas, R. *Arch. Surg.*, 1925, **10**, 293; Boulton, T.B. 'Classical File', *Surv. Anesthesiol.*, 1984, **28**, 150

12. Halsted, W.S. *New York Med. J.*, 1885, **42**, 294; Hall, R.J. *New York Med. J.*, 1884, **40**, 463

13. Braun, H. *Arch. Klin. Chir.*, 1902, **69**, 541

14. Abel, J.J. *Johns Hopkins Hosp. Bull.*, 1897, **8**, 151

15. Crile, G.W. *Cleveland Med. J.*, 1897, **11**, 355

16. Cushing, H.W. *Ann. Surg.*, 1902, **36**, 321

17. Redman, A. In *Hollander Schneidermühl's 'Handbuch des Zahnartzl'*, Heilmittellehre, 1890, p.149

18. Fourneau, E. (1872–1949). In *Bull. Soc. Pharmacol.*, 1904, **10**, 141

19. Einhorn, A. *Münch. Med. Wochenschr.*, 1899, **46**, 1218

20. Braun, H. *Dtsch. Med. Wochenschr.*, 1905, **31**, 1667

21. Rose, W. In *Regional Anaesthesia 1884–1984*, Centennial Meeting of Regional Anaesthesia, edited by D. B. Scott *et al.*, Production ICM AB, Sodertalje, 1984; Rose, W. *Anestheziol. Reanimatol.*, 1982, **1**, 3

22. Uhlmann, T. *Narkose und Anaes.*, 1929, **6**, 168

23. Eisleb, O. *et al. Arch. Exp. Path. u. Phar.*, 1931, **160**, 53

24. Gordh, T. *Anaesthesia*, 1949, **4**, 4

25. Telivuo, L.J. (1923–70). In *Ann. Chir. Gynaecol. Fenn.* **52**, 513; see also Boulton, T.B. 'Classical File', *Surv. Anesthesiol.*, 1991, **35**, 600–620

26. Reynolds, F. *Anaesthesia*, 1993, **46**, 339–340

27. Rynd, F. *Dublin Med. Press*, 1845, **13**, 167; *Dublin J. Med. Sci.*, 1861, **32**, 13

28. Wood, A. *Edinb. Med. Surg. J.*, 1855, **82**, 26; Howard-Jones, N. *J. Hist. Med.* 1947, **2**, 201; Boulton, T.B. *Surv. Anesthesiol.*, 1984, **28**, 346–354

29. See also Schwidetsky, O. *Anesth. Analg. Curr. Res.*, 1944, **23**, 34; Jones, N.H. *J. Hist. Med.*, 1947, **2**, 201

30. Viets, H.R. *Bull. Hist. Med.*, 1935, **3**, 701

31. Magendie, F. *J. Physiol. Exp. Path.*, 1827, **7**, 66

32. von Anrep, B. *Arch. Physiol.*, 1880, **21**, 38

33. Corning, J.L. *New York Med. J.*, 1885, **42**, 483 (reprinted in 'Classical File', *Surv. Anesthesiol.*, 1960, **4**, 332); *Med. Rec. (NY)*, 1888, **33**, 291

34. Corning, J.L. *Local Anesthesia*, Appleton, New York, 1886; see also Little, D.M. 'Classical File', *Surv. Anesthesiol.*, 1979, **23**, 271

35. Quincke, H.I. *Berl. Klin. Wochenschr.*, 1891, **28**, 930; *ibid.*, **25**, 809; *Verh. Kongr. Inn. Med.*, 1891, **10**, 321

36. Wynter, W.E. *Lancet*, 1891, **1**, 981

37. Bier, A. *Zbl. Chir.*, 1892, **19**, 57

38. Bier, A. *Verh. Dtsch. Ges. Chir.*, 1908, **37**, 204

39. Bier, A. *Dtsch. Z. Chir.*, 1899, **51**, 361 (translated and reprinted in 'Classical File', *Surv. Anesthesiol.*, 1962, **6**, 352)

40. Tuffier, T. *C. R. Soc. Biol. (Paris)*, 1899, **51**, 882

41. Tait, F.D. and Caglieri, G.E. *J.A.M.A.*, 1900, **35**, 6

42. Matas, R. *Phil. Med. J.*, 1900, **6**, 882

43. Donitz, A. *Münch. Med. Wochenschr.*, 1903, **50**, 1452; Bier, A. *Verh. Dtsch. Ges. Chir.*, 1905, **34**, 115

44. Fourneau, E. *Bull. Soc. Pharmacol. (Paris)*, 1904, **10**, 141

45. Chaput, H. *Bull. Soc. Chir. (Paris)*, 1904, **NS30**, 835

46. Einhorn, A. *Dtsch. Med. Wochenschr.*, 1905, **31**, 1668

47. Heineke, H. and Läwen, A. *Dtsch. Z. Chir.*, 1905, **80**, 192; Braun, H. *Dtsch. Med. Wochenschr.*, 1905, **31**, 1667

48. Barker, A.E. *Lond. Clin. J.*, 1906, **28**, 4; *Br. Med. J.*, 1907, **1**, 665; *ibid.*, 1908, **1**, 264; **2**, 453; Lee J.A. *Anaesthesia*, 1979, **34**, 885

49. Brownlee, A. *Practitioner*, 1911, Feb., p.214

50. Dean, H.P. *Br. Med. J.*, 1906, **1**, 1086; Akhtar, M. *Anaesthesia*, 1972, **27**, 330

51. Gray, H.T. *Lancet*, 1909, **2**, 913

52. Babcock, W.W. *New York St. J. Med.*, 1914, **50**, 637

53. See also Macintosh, R.R. *Region. Anesth.*, 1978, **1**, 2; Lee, J.A. *Region. Anesth.*, 1985, **10**, 99

54. Labat, G. *Ann. Surg.*, 1921, **74**, 673

55. Pitkin, G.P. *J. Med. Soc. N. J.*, 1927, **24**, 425; *Am. J. Surg.*, 1928, **5**, 537

56. Chen, K.K. and Schmidt, C.F. *J. Pharmacol. Exp. Ther.*, 1924, **24**, 331; *J.A.M.A.*, 1926, **87**, 836

57. Ocherblad, N.F. and Dillon, T.G. *J.A.M.A.*, 1927, **88**, 1135

58. Rudolf, R.D. and Graham, J.D. *Am. J. Med. Sci.*, 1927, **173**, 399

59. Gray, H.T. and Parsons, L. *Q. J. Med.*, 1912, **5**, 339

60. Smith, G.S. and Porter, W.T. *Am. J. Physiol.*, 1915, **38**, 108

61. Jonnesco, T. *Br. Med. J.*, 1909, **2**, 1396

62. Koster, H. *Am. J. Surg.*, 1928, **5**, 554 (reprinted in 'Classical File', *Surv. Anesthesiol.*, 1968, **12**, 306 and *Surv. Anesthesiol.*, 1978, **22**, 301)
63. Keyes, E.L. and McLelland, A.M. *Am. J. Surg.*, 1930, **9**, 1: *J.A.M.A.*, 1931, **96**, 2085
64. Jones, H.W. *Br. J. Anaesth.*, 1930, **7**, 146
65. Kirschner, M. *Surg. Gynecol. Obstet.*, 1932, **55**, 317
66. Sebrechts, J. *Br. J. Anaesth.*, 1934, **12**, 4
67. Wilson, W.E. *Br. J. Anaesth.*, 1934, **11**, 43
68. Lemmon, W.T. *Ann. Surg.*, 1940, **111**, 141
69. Dean, H.P. *Br. Med. J.*, 1907, **2**, 870
70. Sise, L.F. *Surg. Clin. North Am.*, 1935, **15**, 1501 (reprinted in 'Classical File', *Surv. Anesthesiol.*, 1957, **1**, 266)
71. Eisleb, O. *Arch. Exp. Path. Pharmak.*, 1931, **160**, 53
72. Ekblom, L. and Widman, B. *Acta Anaesth. Scand.*, 1966, suppl.23, p.419
73. Cope, R.W. *Anaesthesia*, 1954, **9**, 249; Editorial, *Br. J. Anaesth.*, 1954, **26**, 233
74. Foster Kennedy, G. *et al. Surg. Gynecol. Obstet.*, 1950, **91**, 385 (reprinted in 'Classical File', *Surv. Anesthesiol.*, 1964, **8**, 273)
75. Thorsen, G. *Acta Surg. Scand.*, 1947, suppl.95, p.121
76. Dripps, R.D. and Vandam, L.D. *J.A.M.A.*, 1954, **156**, 1486 (reprinted in 'Classical File', *Surv. Anesthesiol.*, 1970, **14**, 308)
77. Hutter, C.D.D. *Anaesthesia*, 1990, **45**, 859
78. Cathelin, F. *C. R. Soc. Biol. (Paris)*, 1901, **53**, 452
79. Sicard, J.-A. *C. R. Soc. Biol. (Paris)*, 1901, **53**, 396
80. Stoekel, W. *Zbl. Chir.*, 1909, **33**, 1
81. Laewen, A. *Zbl. Chir.*, 1910, **37**, 708
82. Labat, G. *Regional Anesthesia.*, Saunders, Philadelphia, 1923
83. Campbell, M.F. *Am. J. Urol.*, 1933, **30**, 245
84. Hingson, R.A. and Edwards, W.B. *J.A.M.A.*, 1943, **121**, 225
85. Heile, B. *Archiv für Klinische Chirurgie*, 1913, **101**, 845
86. Pagés-Miravé, F. *Revta Sanid. Milit. (Madrid)*, 1921, **11**, 351 (translated and reprinted in 'Classical File', *Surv. Anesthesiol.*, 1961, **5**, 326)
87. Dogliotti, A.M. *Zbl. Chir.*, 1931, **58**, 3141
88. Aburel, E. *Bull. Soc. d'Obstet. Gynaecol. (Paris)*, 1931, **20**, 85
89. Odom, C.B. *Am. J. Surg.*, 1936, **34**, 547
90. Dawkins, C.J.M. *Proc. Roy. Soc. Med.*, 1945, **38**, 299
91. Curbelo, M.M. *Anesth. Analg. Curr. Res.*, 1949, **28**, 13
92. Tuohy, E.B. *Surg. Clin. North Am.*, 1945, **25**, 834
93. Tuohy, E.B. *J.A.M.A.*, 1945, **128**, 262
94. Behar, M., Magori, F., Olshwane, D. and Davidson, J.T. *Lancet*, 1979, **1**, 527
95. Jolly, C. and Lee, J.A. *Anaesthesia*, 1957, **12**, 49
96. Lee, J.A. *Anaesthesia*, 1949, **4**, 169
97. Riha, J. *Anaesthesist*, 1962, **11**, 230
98. Holmes, C.M. *Lancet*, 1963, **1**, 245
99. Armstrong, P., Brockway, M. and Wildsmith, J.A.W. *Anaesthesia*, 1990, **45**, 11
100. Albright, G.A. *Anesthesiology*, **51**, 285

16
Monitoring

Development of measurement in anaesthesia[1]

John Snow placed heavy emphasis on accurate record-keeping, and describes many physical symptoms during anaesthesia. He frequently mentions second- and third-degree anaesthesia, based on observation of signs. In 1848 he records detailed observations in an anaesthetic for a Mrs Brooks, 'the pulse was pretty good',[2] and on 1 November of that year he wrote about a neonate: 'The pulsations of the cord were distinct, but strong and slow. Dashing cold water on the child sometimes caused it to breathe a little sooner, and its lips were black and limbs relaxed. The cord pulsated as far as it was exposed from the vagina – and a little before the placenta was delivered I compressed the cord with my finger and thumb and immediately the breathing became nearly as frequent as natural. When the pressure was removed for a short time the breathing was diminished, but on tying the cord, it improved and the child was soon pretty well.'[3] His clinical notes, incidentally, provide us today with a wealth of historical material about actual patients. Much of the other material of the time is discussion from meetings and descriptions of apparatus.

Mounier, describing the administration of chloroform in 1855, in addition to insisting that wounded patients were kept supine, noted 'an intelligent assistant timed pulse and respiration rates by the second hand of a watch'.[4] Figure 16.1 depicts Joseph Clover (1825–82 – see Chapter 3) in the 1860s with his finger on the pulse of a patient being given chloroform.

In 1864 the Chloroform Committee of the Royal Medical and Chirurgical Society noted that in animal experiments with chloroform, 'the number of respirations is reduced by half and the frequency of the heart's action is increased by an inverse ratio ... the pulse, however, became extremely rapid'.[5] The Nitrous Oxide Committee of 1868 reported 'recommend ... that, when dangerous symptoms appear the exhibition (of anaesthesia) be at once suspended, and, should respiration not take place, artificial respiration

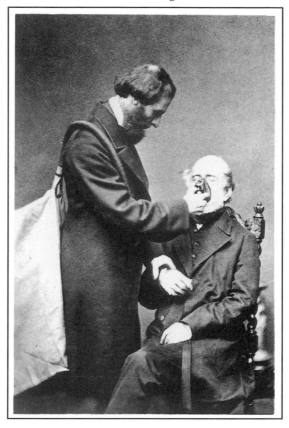

Figure 16.1   Joseph Clover monitoring the patient's pulse

be resorted to'.[6] There is no description of exactly what these dangerous symptoms were, but they imply close observation of the patient's reactions.

At the end of the century, Frederick Hewitt wrote: 'Other modifications have been made to this inhaler ... these makers have also added a feather to the vulcanite facepiece so that the respiration may be observed.'[7] Bigelow recorded his observation (during nitrous oxide anaesthesia) of cyanosis, muscle spasm and absence of patient movement at the turn of the century: 'After several inspirations, the patient's lips and the most vascular part of the tumour began to assume a purple colour. She remained quiet however and in a short time was evidently insensible although the muscles were not perfectly relaxed.'[8]

In 1894 Ernest A. Codman (1869–1940), surgeon, and Harvey Williams Cushing (1869–1939), neurosurgeon and Professor of Surgery at Harvard, developed operative monitoring and record-keeping at the Massachusetts General Hospital from the earlier pioneering work of John Snow and others. Recording of the new skill of arterial pressure measurements was included in the Massachusetts records from 1901.

In 1905 Korotkoff described sphygmomanometric sounds (see p.157), and in 1911 McKesson added respiration rate and inspired oxygen concentration to the monitoring armamentarium. Oximetry was first performed as early as 1913.[9]

Guedel recategorized Snow's stages and clinical signs of anaesthesia in 1920. There was steady development of Einthoven's discovery, the electrocardiogram, which eventually led to its gradual introduction into anaesthetic practice during the early 1960s using cathode ray oscilloscopes. The first nerve stimulator in man to assess neuromuscular function was used by Grob in 1949.[10]

The 1950s saw the widespread exploitation of technology that had been driven forward by World War II. Oxygen analysis with paramagnetic analysers (described by Linus Pauling in 1946[11]) was introduced, and Postoperative monitoring in recovery rooms was advocated by J.Alfred Lee at Southend Hospital, UK. W. N. Rollason,[51] of Aberdeen, advocated the use of intraoperative ECG monitoring in the UK. Oxygen failure warning devices became commonplace on British Oxygen Company anaesthetic machines, e.g. 'bosun' alarms. Capnography was used clinically in the 1960s, although the infrared analyser had first been employed as early as 1865.[12]

The introduction of better materials allowed increasing use of invasive vascular monitoring, e.g. central venous pressure monitoring in the 1960s. Subclavian vein puncture was first described in 1952. Invasive intra-arterial pressure was measured, first by Bourdon gauges, then by transducers to allow measurement of non-pulsatile pressure during cardiopulmonary bypass. From the beginning they were kept from clotting by slow-running infusions of very dilute heparin. In the 1970s Swan–Ganz catheters[13] were used increasingly for the measurement of cardiac output and for mixed venous sampling. Lategola had previously developed the balloon tip in 1953, and Bradley used a pulmonary artery catheter in the very ill in 1964,[14] but Swan and Ganz combined these approaches and described their catheter in 1970. It was a major milestone for the anaesthetist and intensive care physician.

It is noteworthy that cardiac catheterization had been performed in the horse by Chareau and Marey as early as 1855, in the dog by Claude Bernard in 1879, and in man probably by Bleichroder before

1912, who passed a catheter into his own vascular system[15] and then by Forssmann in 1929.[16] Forssmann was a urologist, and was awarded the Nobel prize for this work in 1956.

The 1970s saw the gradual introduction of ventilator disconnection alarms, and neuromuscular monitoring became common in anaesthesia during the 1980s. In 1986 the Harvard standards of minimal monitoring were promoted. (Extradural analgesia was specifically excluded from these standards!) In 1988 the Association of Anaesthetists of Great Britain and Ireland set their first standards of minimal anaesthetic monitoring, closely followed by the Australian minimal monitoring standards.

Measurement of arterial pressure

Stephen Hales (1677–1761) in 1733 was the first to attempt measurement of the blood pressure of animals by direct cannulation of an artery.[17] The mercury manometer was first used to measure blood pressure in 1828 by Poiseuille (1799–1869), the Paris physiologist.[18] In 1834, Herrison,[19] devised a crude instrument to be placed directly over an artery for clinical measurement of blood pressure. Vierordt (1818–84) was the first to estimate the amount of counter-pressure necessary just to obliterate the arterial pulse.[20] Etienne Jules Marey (1830–1904) in 1875 and von Basch (1837–1905) pioneered clinical sphygmomanometry.[21]

Scipione Riva-Rocci (1863–1937) of Turin introduced the blood-pressure cuff in 1896,[22] although the cuff he used was only 5 cm in width. In 1901, von Recklinghausen (1833–1910) drew attention to the importance of the width of the pneumatic cuff to obtain accurate results. E. A. Codman (1869–1940) in 1894 and Harvey Cushing (1869–1939)[23] of Boston advocated the use of blood-pressure readings regularly during anaesthesia. Korotkoff (1874–1920), a Russian physician, in 1905[24] described the sounds heard over an artery at a point just below the compression cuff.[25] The sounds he described are now divided into five phases as the cuff is deflated: intermittent tapping (systolic pressure); onset of quietness (auscultatory gap); louder sounds; sounds become muffled (often taken as diastolic pressure in UK); sounds disappear (often taken as diastolic pressure in USA).

For a full history of blood pressure measurements in anaesthesia, see Calverley, R. K. 'Classical File', *Surv. Anesthesiol*, 1985, **29**, 78.

Oscillotonometry

The original manual method was developed by Von Recklinghausen using the oscillations of a needle to indicate systolic and diastolic

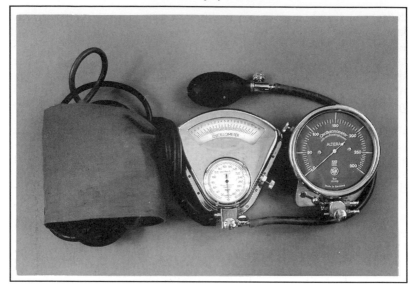

Figure 16.2 Manual oscillotonometers

pressures (Figure 16.2). The automatic oscillotonometers were developed by equipment companies in the 1970s and the pressures, detected by a transducer in the monitor, were analysed and presented as systolic, diastolic and a computed mean arterial pressure. Improvements included artefact rejection (e.g. of surgeons leaning on the cuff during the measurement). The automated oscillotonometer proved accurate and became the standard non-invasive measure of arterial pressure.[26] Monitors using ultrasonic detectors (2–10 MHz), placed over the brachial artery to detect arterial pulsation in a similar way to the transducers above, were less satisfactory as they required more protection from movement. Finger arterial pressure monitors (Finapres)[27] promised a new chapter in non-invasive monitoring as they used a plethysmographic method to indicate continual arterial pressure. Although they have compared well with intra-arterial monitoring,[28] they have not fulfilled their promise.

Central venous pressure

Venous pressures were first measured by Stephen Hales (1677–1761) in 1733 in a mare, and first measured in man by Frey in 1902[29] and used clinically in 1910.[30] Forssmann's pioneering work on cardiac catheterization,[31] and the development of better materials stimulated progress. The first plastic intravenous catheter (polythene) was used in 1945.[32] Central venous catheters developed rapidly after this.[33] Access via veins in the arms did not prove reliable,[34] and the subclavian[35] or internal jugular[36] veins became favoured.

Blood-gas and electrolyte measurements

Blood-gas measurements were started by Pflüger (1829–1910) as early as 1872.[37] Leland Clark developed his polarographic oxygen electrode in 1956,[38] which is the basis of the modern oxygen electrode, although modifications have been produced.[39] At much the same time, the polio epidemic in Copenhagen stimulated methods for measuring arterial P_{CO_2}. At first Astrup measured the pH of blood after tonometry with differing CO_2 concentrations to determine its P_{CO_2}. But the development of the P_{CO_2} electrode was to greatly facilitate this measurement, and a full acid-base picture could be derived from the Siggaard-Andersen nomogram.[40] Today the calculations are performed by microprocessors.

For a full history of this subject, see Astrup, P. and Severinghaus, J. W. *History of Gases, Acids and Bases*, Munksgaard, Copenhagen, 1986.

Flame photometry was pioneered for the measurment of electrolyte concentrations in blood in 1947,[41] and ion-selective electrodes were described in 1963.[42]

Electroencephalogram

The electrical activity of the brain in animals was noted by Richard Caton of Liverpool (1842–1926) in 1875. Hans Berger (1873–1941)[43] in 1931 described alpha rhythms in man. Adrian and Matthews (1934) developed the clinical uses of the electroencephalogram.[44] This technique was first used in anaesthesia in 1950,[45] although it had been suggested by Gibbs in 1937.[46]

Temperature

The founder of clinical thermometry was C. A. Wunderlich (1815–77), Professor of Medicine at Leipzig, whose classic work appeared in 1868:[47] 'Before his work fever was a disease; after it, a symptom' (C. Garrison).

Magnetic resonance imaging

The phenomenon of nuclear magnetic resonance was discovered in 1946,[48] but it was not used for imaging until computing power had advanced sufficiently in 1973.[49] It is now in general clinical use for imaging, and poses various problems for the anaesthetist due to the strong magnetic fields.[50]

References

1. Symposium issue. *Anaesth. Intensive Care*, 1988, **16**, 5–116
2. Ellis, R.H. (ed.) *The Casebooks of Dr John Snow*, Wellcome Institute for the History of Medicine, 1995, p.22
3. Ellis, R.H. (ed.) *The Casebooks of Dr John Snow*, Wellcome Institute for the History of Medicine, 1995, p.30
4. Mounier, C. *C. R. Acad. Sci. Paris*, 1855, **40**, 530
5. *Med-Chir. Trans.*, 1864, **47**, 331
6. *Br. Med. J.*, 1868, **ii**, 622
7. Hewitt, F.W. *Anaesthetics and their Administration*, 1893, Griffin, London, p.197
8. Bigelow, H.J. *Surgical Anaesthesia – Addresses and Other Papers*, 1900, Boston, p.97
9. Cooke, A. and Barcroft, J. *J. Physiol. (Lond.)* 1913, **47**, 35
10. Grob, A. *et al. Bull. Johns Hopkins Hosp.*, 1949, **84**, 279
11. Pauling, L. *Science*, 1946, **103**, 338
12. Tyndal, J. *Trans. Roy. Coll. Surg. Engl.*, 1865, **4**, 139
13. Swan, H.J.C. and Ganz, W. *et al. N. Engl. J. Med.*, 1970, **283**, 447
14. Lategola, M. and Rahn, H. *Proc. Soc. Exp. Biol. Med.*, 1953, **84**, 667; Bradley, R. D. *Lancet*, 1964, **2**, 941
15. Bleichroder, F. *Berl. Klin. Wochenschr.*, 1912, **49**, 1503
16. Forssmann, W.T. *Klin. Wochenschr.*, 1929, **8**, 2085; Harvey A.M. *Science at the Bedside, 1905–1945*, Johns Hopkins University Press, Baltimore, 1981
17. Willius, F.A. and Keyes, T.E. *Cardiac Classics*, Mosby, St Louis, 1941, p.131
18. Poiseuille, J.L.M. *Archs. Gén. Méd. (Paris)*, 1828, **18**, 550
19. Herrison, J. *Le Sphygmométre*, Crochard, Paris, 1834; Clark-Kennedy, A.E. (ed.). *Stephen Hales: Physiologist and Botanist*, Cambridge University Press, 1977; Booth, J. *Proc. Roy. Soc. Med.*, 1977, **70**, 793
20. Vierordt, K. *Arch. Physiol. Heilk.*, 1854, **13**, 284
21. Von Basch, S. Z. *Klin. Med.*, 1883, **33**, 673
22. Riva-Rocci, S. *Gaz. Med. di Torin*, 1896, **47**, 981 (reprinted in English translation in *Foundations of Anesthesiology*, edited by A. Faulconer and T. E. Keys, Thomas, Springfield, Ill, p.1043)
23. Cushing, H.W. *Ann. Surg.*, 1902, **36**, 321; *Boston Med. Surg. J.*, 1903, **148**, 291 (reprinted in 'Classical File', *Surv. Anesthesiol.*, 1960, **4**, 419)
24. Korotkoff, N.S. *Izvest. imp. Vyenno-Med. Acad. St Petersburg*, 1905, **11**, 365
25. Comroe, J.H. *Anesth. Analg. (Cleve.)*, 1976, **55**, 900
26. Friesen, R.H. and Lichtor, J.L. *Anesth. Analg.*, 1981, **60**, 742; Kimble, K.J. *et al. Anesthesiology*, 1981, **54**, 423; Hutton, P. *et al. Anaesthesia*, 1984, **39**, 261
27. Dorlas, J.C. *et al. Anesthesiology*, 1985, **62**, 342

28. Kermode, J.L., Davis, N.J. and Thompson, W.R. *Anaes. and Intensive Care*, 1989, **17**, 470
29. Frey, A. *Dtsch. Arch. Klin. Med.*, 1902, **73**, 511
30. Moritz, F. and von Tabora, D. *Dtsch. Arch. Klin. Med.*, 1910, **98**, 475
31. Forssmann, W. *Münch. Med. Wochenschr*, 1931, **78**, 489
32. Meyers, L. *Am. J. Nurs.*, 1945, **45**, 930
33. Peters, J.L. *Central Venous Catheterization and Parenteral Nutrition*, Wright, Bristol, 1983
34. Johnston, A.O.B. and Clark, R.G. *Lancet*, 1972, **2**, 1395; Mathews, C.A. *Br. Med. J.*, 1973, **1**, 481
35. Yoffa, D. *Lancet*, 1965, **2**, 614
36. English, I.C.W. *et al. Anaesthesia*, 1969, **24**, 521
37. Gothard, J.W.W. *et al. Anaesthesia* 1980, **35**, 890
38. Clark, L.C. *Trans. Am. Soc. Artif. Intern. Organs*, 1956, **2**, 41
39. Laver, M.B. and Seifen, A. *Anesthesiology*, 1965, **26**, 73
40. Siggaard-Andersen, O. *et al. Scand. J. Clin. Lab. Invest.*, 1960, **12**, 177
41. Hald, P.M.J. *Biol. Chem.*, 1947, **167**, 499
42. Friedman, S.M. *et al. J. Appl. Physiol.*, 1963, **18**, 950
43. Berger, H. *Arch. f. Psychiat.*, 1931, **94**, 16
44. Adrian, E.B. and Mathews, B.H.C. *Brain*, 1934, **57**, 355
45. Courtin, R.F. *et al. Proc. Staff Mayo Clin.*, 1950, **25**, 197
46. Gibbs, F.A. and Gibbs, L. *Arch. Intern. Med.*, 1937, **60**, 154
47. Wunderlich, C.A. *Medical Thermometry*, 2nd edn, translated by W.B. Woodman, New Sydenham Society, London, 1871; see also *Br. Med. J.*, 1965, **1**, 1449; Allen, L.G. In *The History of Anaesthesia*, edited by R. S. Atkinson and T. B. Boulton, Royal Society of Medicine, London, 1989, pp.368–371
48. Purcell, E.M. *et al.* and Bloch, F. *et al. Phys. Rev.*, 1946, **69**, 37, 127
49. Lauterbur, P. *Nature*, 1973, **242**, 190
50. Menon, D.K. *et al.* and Peden, C.J. *et al. Anaesthesia*, 1992, **47**, 240, 508
51. Rollason, W.N. *Electrocardiography for the Anaesthetist*, 1st edn, Alden Press, Oxford, 1964

17

Induced hypotension and hypothermia

Ischaemia during surgery

In the early days, deep chloroform anaesthesia was used in an effort (often very successfully) to reduce bleeding. Snow records many ischaemic events in his casebooks, some of which appear to be simply a result of haemorrhage.

Controlled arteriotomy followed by autotransfusion had a vogue in the mid-twentieth century.[1] This was haemorrhagic hypotension, and was often associated with reduced oxygen delivery to the brain and heart and with metabolic acidosis. A better understanding of the physiological principles resulted in the method being rapidly dropped from use.

High intradural spinal analgesia was the method used by Griffiths and Gillies in 1948.[2] High extradural spinal analgesia was tried by Bromage in 1951,[3] with some success, but with both methods removal of sympathetic drive (especially to the heart from the upper four thoracic segments) produced serious instability of the circulation.

At about the same time, hypotension was induced with ganglion-blocking agents. Ganglion-blocking effects were demonstrated for hexamethonium and also for pentamethonium, used to reverse the actions of decamethonium.[4] Useful clinical hypotension was shown to follow pentamethonium.[5] Hexamethonium was preferred to pentamethonium by Hunter,[6] while pentolinium was used by Enderby.[7] Trimetaphan was developed by Sarnoff,[8] and by Magill and others[9] in the early 1950s, although it had been described by Randall and others[10] in 1949. Phenactropinium was later used by Robertson and others.[11]

Of the direct-acting vasodilators, sodium nitroprusside had been used to control hypertensive crises in 1929,[12] and to reduce bleeding during anaesthesia in 1962.[13] It was first deliberately used to produce ischaemia in Britain in 1968.[14] Another direct vasodilator, nitroglycerin (glyceryl trinitrate), was first used for the treatment of angina by William Murrell (1853–1912) of London, in 1879,[15] and found a particular place in control of hypertension after cardiac and other vascular surgery. Labetalol was first used in anaesthesia by Scott *et al.* in 1976.[16]

The influence of the head-up posture on the production of hypotension was demonstrated early on by Enderby and was named 'postural ischaemia' by Sir Henry Dale after watching Enderby at work in 1949. The term 'physiological trespass', to describe the deliberate decrease in the safety margins that is inherent in hypotensive anaesthesia, was coined by John Gillies of Edinburgh.[17]

The plastic surgeon Sir Archibald McIndoe gave induced hypotension his influential support in its early days. Halothane was advocated for hypotension in 1960.[18] Propranolol, used to control the tachycardia seen during hypotension, was a very welcome addition to the therapeutic armamentarium.[19] It enabled the anaesthetist to control the compensatory response of the patient, in particular the young patient (often female) in whom hypotension was considered appropriate for plastic surgical procedures.

This technique has declined in use in the 1990s, partly because of better quality operative techniques, as in otolaryngology and plastic surgery, and partly because in neurosurgery the outcome is considered to be better when it is not used. The risks of induced hypotension are now perceived very often to outweigh the advantages.

See also Verner, I. In *Hypotensive Anaesthesia*, edited by G. E. H. Enderby, Churchill Livingstone, Edinburgh and London, 1985.

Induced hypothermia[20]

The use of deliberate body cooling during cardiac surgery dates from the work of Bigelow and colleagues in Toronto in 1950.[21] They pointed out that a hypothermic dog (25°C) would survive exclusion of the heart from the circulation for 15 min, whereas a normothermic dog would survive only 5–9 min. With progressive cooling, rectal temperature and oxygen consumption showed an almost linear relationship, but it was of fundamental importance to prevent shivering as even slight shivering could double oxygen consumption. No oxygen debt was incurred by the tissues. The effects of hypothermia were well described by Churchill-Davidson.[22]

The use of hypothermia to close an atrioseptal defect under direct vision was reported in 1953.[23] In the same year Swan used hypothermia in 15 patients with occlusion of the circulation for between

2 and 9.5 min with only one operative death.[24] In Britain, hypothermia was much used in open heart surgery by Broom and Sellick.[25] (See also Chapter 12.)

Hypothermia was produced by surface cooling (slow) or by direct blood cooling using an arteriovenous shunt. Its main use was to allow relatively quick operations on the heart while the circulation was interrupted. It also had a vogue in neurosurgery for the treatment of aneurysms. One complication was the possibility of air embolism. The development of pump oxygenators allowed more time for surgical procedures, so that deliberate hypothermia became superseded.

Falls in body temperature associated with anaesthesia have been recorded since the beginning of the century.[26] In recent times it has been associated with prolonged surgery, often with large volume replacements of blood or blood substitutes.[27] There is also a greater risk in paediatric patients.[28]

References

1. Gardner, W.J. *J.A.M.A.*, 1946, **132**, 572 (reprinted in 'Classical File', *Surv. Anesthesiol.*, 1969, **13**, 220)
2. Koster, H. *Am. J. Surg.*, 1928, **5**, 554; Vehrs, G.R. *N. W. Med. Seattle*, 1931, **30**, 256, 322; Griffiths, M.W.C. and Gillies, J. *Anaesthesia*, 1948, **3**, 134 (reprinted in 'Classical File', *Surv. Anesthesiol.*, 1980, **24**, 342)
3. Bromage, P.R. *Anaesthesia*, 1951, **6**, 26
4. Paton, W.D.M. and Zaimis, E.J. *Nature*, 1948, **162**, 810
5. Organe, G.S.W. *et al. Lancet*, 1949, **1**, 21
6. Hunter, A.R. *Lancet*, 1950, **1**, 251; Shackleton, R.P.W. *Br. Med. J.*, 1951, **1**, 1054; Wyman, J.B. *Proc. Roy. Soc. Med.*, 1953, **46**, 605
7. Enderby, G.E.H. *Lancet*, 1950, **1**, 1145; Enderby, G.E.H. and Pelmore, J.F. *Lancet*, 1951, **1**, 663; Enderby, G.E.H. *Lancet*, 1954, **2**, 1097
8. Sarnoff, S.J. *et al. Circulation*, 1952, **6**, 63
9. Magill, I.W. *et al. Lancet*, 1953, **1**, 219
10. Randall, L.O. *et al. J. Pharmacol. Exp. Ther.*, 1949, **97**, 48
11. Robertson, J.D. *et al. Br. J. Anaesth.*, 1957, **29**, 342
12. Johnson, C.C. *Arch. Int. Pharmacodyn. Thér.*, 1929, **35**, 480
13. Moraca, P. *et al. Anesthesiology*, 1962, **23**, 193
14. Jones, G.O.M. and Cole, P. *Br. J. Anaesth.*, 1968, **40**, 804
15. Murrell, W. *Lancet*, 1879, **2**, 80
16. Scott, D.B. *et al. Br. J. Clin. Pharmacol.*, 1976, suppl. 817
17. Gillies, J. *Ann. Roy. Coll. Surg.*, 1950, **7**, 204
18. Enderby, G.E.H. *Anaesthesia*, 1960, **15**, 25
19. Hellewell, J. and Potts, M.W. *Br. J. Anaesth.*, 1966, **38**, 794; Johnstone, M. *Br. J. Anaesth.*, 1966, **38**, 516
20. Holdcroft, A. *Body Temperature Control.*, Baillière Saunders, London, 1980

21. Bigelow, W.G., Lindsay, W.K., Harrison, R.C. and Gordon, R.A. *Am. J. Surg.*, 1950, **160**, 125; Bigelow, W.G., Callaghan, J.C. and Hopps, J.A. *Ann. Surg.*, 1950, **132**, 531

22. Churchill-Davidson, H.C. *Br. J. Anaesth.*, 1955, **27**, 313; see also Scurr C.F. *Proc. Roy. Soc. Med.*, 1955, **48**, 1077; Lucas, B.G.B. *Proc. Roy. Soc. Med.*, 1956, **49**, 345; Brock, R. *Proc. Roy. Soc. Med.*, 1956, **49**, 347; Delorme, E.J. *Anaesthesia*, 1956, **11**, 221

23. Lewis, F.J. and Taufig, M. *Surgery*, 1953, **33**, 52

24. Swan, H., Zeavin, I., Blount, S.G. and Virtue, R.W. *J. Am. Med. Ass.*, 1953, **153**, 1081

25. Broom, B. and Sellick, B.A. *Lancet*, 1955, **2**, 452–455

26. Morley, W.H. *Am. Gynecol.*, 1903, **3**, 300

27. Rees, J.R. *Lancet*, 1958, **1**, 556; Vale, R.J. and Lunn, H.F. *Proc. Roy. Soc. Med.*, 1958, **1**, 556; Searle, J.F. *Br. J. Anaesth.*, 1971, **43**, 1095; Newman, B.J. *Anaesthesia*, 1971, **26**, 177

28. Calvert, D.G. *Anaesthesia*, 1962, **17**, 29

18

Resuscitation, postoperative and intensive care

Resuscitation[1]

Expired air ventilation has been used throughout history in an effort to revive the apparently dead.[2] Tracheostomy was performed in the twelfth and thirteenth centuries in the treatment of drowned persons. Paracelsus (1493–1541) is usually credited with the introduction of the bellows to ventilate the lungs.

The modern history of resuscitation begins in the middle of the eighteenth century. This was a period when a wave of humanitarianism spread through Europe. A Society for the Recovery of Drowned Persons was founded in Amsterdam in 1767. In Germany, early attempts at resuscitation were made by Langenbuch, Koenig and Maass.[3] In Britain the Humane Society, later the Royal Humane Society, was established by William Hawes in 1774. Classic early contributions to the literature include those of John Hunter (1718–83)[4] in 1776, Kite[5] in 1788 and Herholdt and Rafn in 1796.[6]

Artificial ventilation of the lungs was advocated by Marshall Hall (1790–1857)[7] in 1856, the discoverer of reflex action, who described a method of rotating the patient's body combined with pressure on the back to aid expiration. Silvester (1818–1902)[8] described his method in 1858, and Holger Nielsen[9] published details of a new technique in 1932. In the same year, Eve (1871–1952) introduced the tilting board method.[10] Artificial respiration by direct laryngeal intubation with a modified O'Dwyer's tube was performed by Rudolph Matas of New Orleans in 1902.[11]

Reports of deaths during anaesthesia, in the years following 1846, led to interest in the study of cardiac arrest. Ventricular fibrillation was first described by MacWilliam of Aberdeen in 1887.[12] The first successful internal cardiac massage was probably performed in Norway in 1901[13] and by Beck in 1947.[14] The first in Britain was reported by Starling (1866–1927)[15] in 1902. Beck[16] successfully defibrillated the human heart in 1937. The first external defibrillation of the human heart was in 1956.[17] External cardiac compression became popular following the work of Kouwenhoven and others in 1960.[18] The first successful cardiopulmonary resuscitation outside the operating theatre was undertaken by Beck in 1956.[19]

Postoperative care

Postoperative observation or recovery rooms[20]

In 1863, Florence Nightingale, who had founded the school of nursing at St.Thomas's Hospital three years before, described an area set apart for patients following operations. However, it was nearly a century later that the first formal postoperative observation room in the UK was opened. They had been advocated by A. L. Flemming, President of the Anaesthetic Section of the Medical Institute of Birmingham in 1921,[21] and instituted in the USA in 1923. Lundy at the Mayo Clinic organized a similar facility there in 1942. Lowenthal and Russell's paper of 1951 had an important influence on the spread of such units in the USA,[22] where their advantages were realized sooner than in the UK.

Amongst the first postoperative observation wards (recovery wards) opened in the UK was that at East Grinstead (first used in 1946, for the particular problems arising after plastic surgery, where 10 single-bedded glass-fronted rooms were placed adjacent to the operating theatres),[23] and that opened in 1955 by J.Alfred Lee at Southend Hospital. The latter had four beds, was staffed 24 hours a day, and was a development that was fiercely opposed by some surgeons.[24] We are influenced nowadays by recommendations for standards of postoperative care from professional bodies, for example those issued in 1988 by The American Society of Anesthesiologists.[25] Similar recommendations have been issued by the Association of Anaesthetists in London.

Intensive care[26]

The significance of this development was that, for the first time, anaesthetists stepped out of the operating theatres and developed their own wards for the care of their patients. They often had a hard battle with colleagues to obtain space, equipment and staff for the intensive care of critically ill patients. It was their skills in the areas of mechanical ventilation and circulatory support which were of life-saving benefit to the seriously ill patients of that time. Against this background, a chronological view of the way in which intensive care has developed is presented here:

1801   Five two-bedded rooms, reserved for patients who were dangerously ill or who had undergone a major operation (the other bed being occupied at night by a nurse), were planned for the renovation of the Forth Banks Infirmary, Newcastle upon Tyne, UK.[27]

1885   Joseph O'Dwyer (1841–98), a physician in New York, invented a short metal endotracheal tube as a life-saving alternative to tracheostomy in diphtheria. The upper flange prevented it falling through the larynx.

1888   O'Dwyer combined his tube with George Fell's (1850–1918) (from Buffalo, New York) resuscitation bellows for intermittent positive pressure ventilation (IPPV). He later added a cuff to his tube. The apparatus was used for treating respiratory arrest and for the relief of upper airway obstruction as caused by diphtheria, and later for thoracic anaesthesia.

1929   Drinker developed the tank ventilator in which the patient's body (usually those paralysed by poliomyelitis) was intermittently subjected to negative pressure, causing respiration. The patient's head was outside the tank.[28] These were large, awkward devices which severely restricted nursing access. An attempt was made to solve some of these problems with the 'see-saw' rocking-bed respirators.

1934   Leslie Cole of Cambridge used curare in the treatment of tetanus.[29]

1938   In Britain there was an epidemic of poliomyelitis with a higher than usual incidence of cases suffering respiratory paralysis. The Drinker apparatus was expensive and made nursing care cumbersome. Moreover there were not enough available for the needs of the epidemic. Edward Thomas Both (1908–87) was an Australian who happened to be in London at this time. He and his brother Don had developed the world's first commercial direct writing electrocardiogram in 1932 and he was in Britain to promote it. The Both company designed a simple inexpensive apparatus, made largely of plywood (though still called an iron lung) and suitable for rapid manufacture. Lord Nuffield heard of this and announced that he was prepared to manufacture up to 5000 Both respirators in his factory in Cowley, Oxford. Moreover he would give one or more to any hospital in the British Empire which requested one. As many as 1800 were built before the outbreak of World War II in 1939. Both was awarded the OBE in recognition of his work.

1940s   The respiratory care unit was founded at Oxford.[30]

1942   The development of non-depolarizing neuromuscular block-ing agents by Griffith produced the need for new ventilators for anaesthesia which could be combined with the new endotracheal techniques of Magill and Macintosh, which were more convenient for the operating theatre environment and also solving the problem of oropharyngeal and gastric secretions entering the trachea.[31]

1950s   This decade saw the appearance of intensive care units as we now know them. 'The concept of intensive therapy was founded and formulated when the patient was brought to the anaesthesiolo-gist for treatment and not vice versa'.[32]

1952   The poliomyelitis epidemic which occurred in Copenhagen in 1952 had enormous influence on the development of care of patients with respiratory failure.[33] Bjørn Ibsen (1915–)* was called in by Professor Lassen to help with the ventilatory management of polio patients in the Blegdam Hospital. He developed the method of hand ventilation through a tracheostomy tube (Figure 18.1), and an understanding of the importance of carbon dioxide levels. Almost the whole of the student body of the medical school were required to help with manual ventilation, and teaching activities were sus-pended until the epidemic was over. Ibsen also realized the impor-tance of treating the patient early, before admission to hospital, the

---

* **Bjørn Ibsen (1915–)**

Worked under H. K. Beecher in Boston, Mass. in 1949, returning to Denmark in 1950 to work freelance at the University Hospital in Copenhagen until 1953. In 1952 the poliomyelitis epidemic occurred. Interested in measurement of carbon dioxide concentrations in air.[34] Also in communication with Bower in Los Angeles who had achieved significant reductions in mortality from bulbar poliomyelitis. Thus when he was called in by Professor Lassen to discuss management of cases in the current Danish epidemic, he used his knowledge first to manage a sick 12–year-old patient with paralysis by artificial ventilation through a tracheostomy with success, and later to use carbon dioxide measurement to assess the degree of ventilation required. As the number of bulbar poliomyelitis cases continued to increase it became possible to outline the principles of treatment, and patients with respiratory impairment were transferred to a special department in the Blegdam Hospital. Problems arose because of a deterioration of patients during transfer to the hospital, and it was realized that treatment had to begin before transfer if respiration was impaired.

In 1953, started to work in the Kommunehospital (or Municipal Hospital) of Copenhagen. Within a few months a recovery room with 10 beds was opened. In 1954 he was appointed head of a newly established department of anaesthesiology, and was able to continue his work on intensive therapy. Within 5 years he was able to report on the management of 259 cases.[37]

Interested in many aspects of the anaesthetists' work, including the use of monitoring equipment and the treatment of chronic pain. In 1974 he published a survey of 1000 consecutive patients treated in his pain clinic.[35]

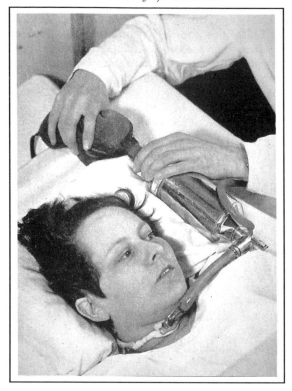

Figure 18.1   Manual ventilation via tracheostomy

anaesthetist going out as part of the ambulance team.[36] The Copen-hagen experience resulted in the development of ventilators in many European countries and in the USA.

Ibsen called his unit the Intensive Therapy Unit. Thus the concept of intensive therapy arose first from experience in respiratory care units when patients suffering from respiratory failure secondary to bulbar poliomyelitis and other neurological diseases required assisted ventilation, and only secondly from the experience of anaesthetists working in postoperative care when the 'intensive care' given during surgery itself was extended for some hours or even days into the postoperative period. Experience gained over many years in resuscitation also proved important. In 1953 Ibsen moved to the Kommunehospital as Chief Anaesthesiologist, where he established a department of intensive therapy with T. Kvittingen, publishing a survey of the first 5 years' work on 259 patients in 1958.[37]

The Copenhagen experience also stimulated interest in blood-gas measurement. The early development of blood gas and blood acid-base measurements have been described by Astrup.[38] Early medical workers with an interest in acid-base disorders included O'Shaughnessy, an Irishman who practised in London during the cholera epidemic of 1831–32.[39] Real progress came in 1912 when Hasselbalch used Sørensen's hydrogen electrode to measure pH in blood.[40] The Copenhagen epidemic led to new analytical developments. The equilibration method was introduced, based on electrometric measuring of pH samples of capillary blood before and after equilibration at two known carbon dioxide tensions.

1953 The Seldinger technique of guidewires to aid insertion of central venous lines.

1954 The Respiratory Unit at Oxford led by Crampton Smith, Spalding and Ritchie Russell was influential in the care of patients suffering from polio (Figure 18.2).[41] It had a strong neurological bias. In Britain, intensive therapy units developed from such respiratory units. Anaesthetists gradually became involved because of their knowledge of respiratory physiology and of ventilation of the lungs and their experience of care of patients during long surgical operations, especially in support of the circulation and of fluid balance. Also, anaesthetists did not own beds, so that other physicians and surgeons did not feel obliged to hand over their patients.

1960s Coronary care units were set up widely in the UK and USA, with associated development of respiratory care units for IPPV of those patients who were also suffering from acute and reversible respiratory failure.

1961 Roger Manley described the Manley Ventilator which did much to enable widespread and easy IPPV. It was relatively cheap, extremely reliable, and was reasonably flexible. It was designed to minimize the the cardiovascular effects of IPPV on the anaesthetized patient; to provide the anaesthetist with as as much information as possible about the ventilation and the degree of relaxation of the patient, thus compensating for the loss of contact with 'the bag'; to be sufficiently small to stand on an anaesthetic machine; and to be powered by gas pressure.[42]

Other examples of early ventilators include the Beaver[43] and the Radcliffe[44] in Britain, the Bang in Denmark in 1953, the Engström in Sweden in 1954, the Mörch Piston ventilator in the USA in 1954 and the Dräger Poliomat in Germany in 1955.

1962 The Department of Health in the UK developed the concept of progressive patient care: 'The systematic grouping of patients

---

**ARTIFICIAL RESPIRATION
BY INTERMITTENT POSITIVE PRESSURE
IN POLIOMYELITIS AND OTHER DISEASES**

A. CRAMPTON SMITH
M.B. Edin., D.A.
ANÆSTHETIST

J. M. K. SPALDING
M.A., D.M. Oxfd, M.R.C.P.
RESEARCH ASSISTANT, DEPARTMENT OF NEUROLOGY

W. RITCHIE RUSSELL
C.B.E., M.A. Oxfd, M.D. Edin., F.R.C.P., F.R.C.P.E.
NEUROLOGIST

RADCLIFFE INFIRMARY, OXFORD

Figure 18.2   Early British publication of respiratory care

according to the degree of their illness and dependence on the nurse, rather than by classification of disease or sex.' Examples given were domiciliary care; long-term care; self-care in hospital; intermediate care in hospital; and the intensive therapy unit (ITU).[45] The basic concepts considered were those of size and space of the unit (as large as 2–5% of hospital beds), the types of patient suitable for ITU care, and the need for standing advisory committees to decide in the event of a disagreement over patient selection (common in those early days). Examples of early units include those run by Spalding (neurologist) and Crampton Smith (anaesthetist) in Oxford, Robinson (anaesthetist) and Sherwood-Jones (physician) in Whiston,[46] Liverpool, and Howells and Hunter (anaesthetist) in Manchester.

1964   At the Birmingham Accident Hospital in the UK, a 'tracheostomy unit' was set up for victims of major trauma, and IPPV was immediately part of the available therapy. What followed was a progressive process of addressing the further problems encountered in ventilating sick and septic patients. For example, the need for humidifiers was immediately apparent. Vascular monitoring and support were then required, and borrowed heavily from the technologies springing up in open heart surgery and cardiopulmonary bypass. The consequence of this collaboration, and the fact that managing ventilators was regarded as a skill most understood by anaesthetists, was that anaesthetists were the originators of most of the fledgling intensive care units in Europe.

1967 The guidelines about intensive care units issued by the British Medical Association were a catalyst in the rapid growth of the subspeciality,[47] at a time of increased hospital building in Europe, Scandinavia, Australia and the USA.

1967 The introduction of positive end-expiratory pressure which often improved oxygenation during IPPV of sick patients, although at the expense of reduced cardiac output.

The end of the 1960s saw the rising popularity of parenteral nutrition for the sick patients who were unable to feed themselves.[48] Parenteral nutrition was not new, having had a few dedicated protagonists starting from the late nineteenth century, including Hodder,[49] Yamakawa[50] and Cuthbertson.[51]

1970 The Intensive Care Society in the UK was founded by Dr Alan Gilston. It was a much needed forum for sharing and debating the difficult issues of this subspeciality. The European Society of Intensive Care was formed later by Dr J.-L. Vincent.

The Fourth World Congress of Anaesthesiologists was held in London and contained a Symposium on Intensive Therapy Units at which many of the leading practitioners of that time took part.[52] Apart from the British Medical Association Planning Unit Report,[47] other influential publications around this time included the Hospital Building Note – Intensive Therapy Unit, No. 27, London, HMSO, 1970. Acceptable criteria were now available which enabled a steady increase in the provision of units in district general hospitals in Britain.

Harold J. C. Swan and William Ganz (cardiologists in Los Angeles) developed balloon-tipped pulmonary artery catheters.[53]

1973 High-frequency jet ventilation was introduced.

1975 The therapeutic intervention scoring system was devised.[54]

1981 Knaus and co-workers invented and later developed APACHE scoring.[55] The shortcomings of this system have more recently been pointed out.[56]

1983 The simplified Acute Physiology Score described.[57] Sepsis score described.[58]

1986 Intensive care nursing was given the recognition it deserved in the UK, due to the convincing arguments of patient dependency scoring.[59] It was also claimed that such nursing was not stressful![60]

1988   The Association of Anaesthetists of Great Britain and Ireland highlighted the provision and problems of intensive care.[61] This was followed by a similar report from the King's Fund in 1989.[62] A UK audit of intensive care at this time showed that 85% were run by anaesthetists. Safe methods of transfer of patients between units was emphasized in the UK.[63] Many European countries have developed comprehensive systems for this.

The 1980s also saw the development of renal support in the intensive care units, using dialysis and filtration techniques.

1991   The Association of Anaesthetists of Great Britain and Ireland published an important document on high-dependency units.[64] There has been a rise of interest in these units for short-term care and monitoring of patients with unstable physiology. They are not generally seen as a place where the longer term treatment of organ failure should take place.

Intensive care units have become central to the function of larger hospitals, including district general hospitals, which take any patients from their local community, however ill they may be, and then may act as a staging post for later transfer to specialist units.

Recent developments in the UK have been recognition of the needs for recognized training programmes and of a career structure for doctors wishing to specialize in intensive therapy (cf. the founding of the College of Surgeons and the Association of Anaesthetists). Intercollegiate committees have been in existence for some years with the aim of providing solutions to these problems, including the possible creation of a diploma to signify completion of training. In other countries, developments have proceeded on different lines. Australia has held a separate fellowship for those wishing to practise intensive therapy. There is also a European Diploma in Anaesthesiology and Intensive Care.[65]

References

1. For a history of resuscitation in the nineteenth century, see McLellan, I. *Anaesthesia*, 1981, **36**, 307; see also Little, D.M. *History of Resuscitation*. 'Classical File', *Surv. Anesthesiol.*, 1981, **25**, 415
2. *Holy Bible.*, II Kings 4: 34–35
3. Böhrer, H. and Goerig, M. *Anaesthesia*, 1995, **50**, 969–971
4. Hunter, J. *Phil. Trans.*, 1776, **66**, 412
5. Kite, C. *An Essay on the Recovery of the Apparently Dead.*, Dilly, London, 1788
6. Herholdt, J.D. and Rafn, C.G. *Life Saving Measures for Drowning Persons*, Copenhagen (reprinted by Scandinavian Society of Anaesthesiologists, Aarhus, 1960)
7. Marshal Hall, M. *Lancet*, 1856, **1**, 229; Ellis, R. *Lancet*, 1868, **2**, 538
8. Silvester, H.R. *Br. Med. J.*, 1858, **2**, 576

9. Nielsen, H. *Ugeskr. Laeg.*, 1932, **94**, 1201

10. Eve, F.C. *Lancet*, 1932, **2**, 995

11. Matas, R. *Am. Med.*, 1902, **3**, 97 (reprinted in 'Classical File', *Surv. Anesthesiol.*, 1978, **22**, 401)

12. Correspondence. *Br. Med. J.*, 1985, **290**, 1985 *et seq.*

13. Keen, W.W. *Ther. Gaz.*, 1904, **28**, 217

14. Beck, C.S. *et al. J.A.M.A.*, 1947, **135**, 985

15. Starling, E.A. *Lancet*, 1902, **2**, 1397 (reprinted in 'Classical File', *Surv. Anesthesiol.*, 1975, **19**, 497)

16. Beck, C.S. and Mautz, F.R. *Ann. Surg.*, 1937, **106**, 525

17. Zoll, P.M. and Paul, M.H. *Circulation*, 1956, **14**, 745

18. Kouwenhoven, W.B. *et al. J.A.M.A.*, 1960, **173**, 1064

19. Beck, C.S. *et al. J.A.M.A.*, 1956, **161**, 434

20. See also Ruth, H.S. *et al, J.A.M.A.*, 1947, **35**, 881 Zuck, D. *Anaesthesia*, 1995, **50**, 435–438

21. Flemming, A.L. *Lancet*, 1923, **2**, 227

22. Lowenthal, P.J. and Russell A.S. *Anesthesiology*, 1951, **12**, 470–476

23. Davies, R.M. and Hunter, J.T. *Lancet*, 1952, **1**, 865–868

24. Jolly, C. and Lee, J.A. *Anaesthesia*, 1957, **12**, 49; Discussion. *Proc. Roy. Soc. Med.*, 1958, **51**, 151; Atkinson, R.S. In *Recent Advances in Anaesthesia and Analgesia: 13*, edited by C. L. Hewer and R. S. Atkinson, Churchill Livingstone, Edinburgh, 1979; Lee, J.A. and Jefferies, M. *The Hospitals of Southend*, Phillimore, Chichester, 1986

25. *Standards for postanesthesia care.*, The American Society of Anesthesiologists, 515 Busse Highway, Park Ridge, Ill., 1988

26. Stoddart, J.C. The history and development of intensive therapy. *Curr. Anaesth. Crit. Care*, 1994, **5**, 115–120

27. Clark, J. *An account of the plan for the internal improvement and extension of the Infirmary at Newcastle*, Edward Walker, Newcastle, 1801, p.13

28. Drinker, P. and McKhann, C.F. *J.A.M.A.*, 1929, **92**, 1658–1660

29. Cole, L. *Lancet*, 1934, **2**, 47–57; Horton, J.M. In *Proceedings 3rd International Congress on History of Anaesthesia*, Wood Library-Museum of Anesthesiology, Park Ridge, Ill., 1992, p.262 (reprinted in 'Classical File', *Surv. Anesthesiol.*, 1995, **39**, 337–338)

30. Smith, A.C. The respiration unit. In *The Nuffield Department of Anaesthetics, Oxford, 1937–62*, edited by R. Bryce-Smith, J. V. Mitchell and J. V. Parkhouse, Oxford University Press, 1963, pp. 52–53

31. Griffith, H.R. and Johnson, G.E. *Anesthesiology*, 1942, **3**, 418 (reprinted in 'Classical File', *Surv. Anesthesiol.*, 1957, **1**, 174)

32. Ibsen, B. *Progress in Anaesthesiology* (Proceedings of the Fourth World Congress of Anaesthesiologists), 1968, edited by T. B. Boulton *et al.*, Excerpta Medica Foundation, Amsterdam, 1970, p.477

33. Wackers, G.L. *Acta Anaesthesiol. Scand.*, 1994, **38**, 419–431

34. Engell, H.C. and Ibsen, B. *Acta Chir. Scand.*, 1952, **104**, 313–328

35. Ibsen, B. *Månedskr. prakt. Lægegern*, 1974, **2**

36. Everberg, G. and Ibsen, B. *Ugeskr. Laegg.*, 1954, **116**, 1077–1078

37. Ibsen, B. and Kvittingen, T.D. *Nord. Med.*, 1958, **60**, 1349

38. Astrup, P. The early development of blood gas and blood acid-base measurements. In *Anaesthesia: Essays on its History*, edited by J. Rupreht *et al.*, Springer-Verlag, Berlin, 1985, pp.176–183
39. O'Shaughnessy, W.B. *Lancet*, 1831–32, **1**, 366
40. Hasselbalch, K.A. *Biochem. Z.*, 1916, **74**, 56–62
41. Crampton Smith, A., Hill, E.E. and Hopson, J.A. *Br. Med. J.*, 1956, **2**, 550
42. Manley, R. *Anaesthesia*, 1961, **16**, 317–323
43. Beaver, R.A. *Lancet*, 1953, **1**, 977
44. Russell, W.R., Schuster, E., Smith, A.C. and Spalding, J.M.K. *Lancet*, 1956, **1**, 539
45. Progressive patient care: interim report of a departmental working group. *Monthly Bull. MOH and PHLS*, 1962, **21**, 218–226
46. A unit for intensive patient care. *Lancet*, 1964, **1**, 657; Robinson, J.S. *Br. J. Anaesth.*, 1966, **38**, 132–142
47. *Intensive Care*. BMA Planning Unit No.1, London, 1967
48. Irving, M.H. and Rushman, G.B. *Anaesthesia*, 1971, **26**, 450–467
49. Hodder, E.M. *Practitioner*, 1873, **10**, 14
50. Yamakawa, S. *Nippon Naika Gakkwai Zasshi*, (1920) **17**, 1
51. Cuthbertson, D.P. *Biochem. J.*, 1930, **24**, 1244
52. Boulton, T.B. *et al.* (eds) *Progress in Anaesthesiology.*, Excerpta Medica, Amsterdam, 1970, pp.477–491
53. Swan, H.J.C. and Ganz, W. *et al.* *N. Engl. J. Med.*, 1970, **283**, 447
54. Cullen, D.J., Civetta, J.M., Briggs, B.A. *et al.* *Crit.Care Med.*, 1975, **2**, 57–61
55. Knaus, W.A., Zimmerman, J.E., Wagner, D.P. *et al.* *Crit. Care Med.*, 1981, **9**, 591–603; Knaus, W.A., Draper, E.A., Wagner, D.P. *et al.* *Crit. Care Med.*, 1985, **13**, 818–829; Zimmerman, J.E. *Crit. Care Med.*, 1989, **17**, suppl.169
56. Cerra, F.B., Negro, F. and Abrams, J. *Arch. Surg.*, 1990, **125**, 519; Civetta, J.M., Hudson-Civetta, J.A., Kirton, O. *et al.* *Surg. Obs. Gyn.*, 1992, **175**, 195–203
57. Le Gall, J.R., Loirat, P., Alperovitch, A. *et al.* *Crit. Care Med.*, 1984, **12**, 975–978
58. Elebute, E.A. and Stoner, H.B. *Br. J. Surg.*, 1983, **70**, 29–31
59. Ball, J. and Oreschnick, R. *Senior Nurse*, 1986, **5**, 30–32
60. Nichols, K.A., Springford, V. and Searle J. *J. Adv. Nursing*, 1981, **6**, 311–315; Eisendrath, S.J., Link, N. and Matthay, M. *Crit. Care Med.*, 1986, **14**, 95–98
61. *Intensive Care Services: Provision for the Future*, Association of Anaesthetists of Great Britain and Ireland, London, 1988
62. *Intensive Care in the United Kingdom.*, King's Fund Panel. *Anaesthesia*, 1989, **44**, 428–431
63. Wright, I.H., McDonald, J.C., Rogers, P.N. and Ledingham, I.McA. *Br. Med. J.*, 1988, **296**, 543–545; Purdie, J.A.M., Ridley, S.A. and Wallace, P.G.M. *Br. Med. J.*, 1990, **300**, 79–81
64. *The High Dependency Unit–Acute Care in the Future*, Association of Anaesthetists of Great Britain and Ireland, London, 1991
65. Stoddart, J.C. *Curr. Anaesth. Crit. Care*, 1994, **5**, 115–120

19

The management of pain

Acute postoperative pain

The management of acute postoperative pain using opium and alcohol was established well before anaesthesia, but is rarely mentioned in the 1840s and 1850s. In 1863 James Paget of St. Bartholomew's Hospital recommended $\frac{1}{4}$ to $\frac{1}{2}$ grain of morphia injected subcutaneously after amputation before return to consciousness.[1] The following year Nussbaum gave 1 grain of intra-operative morphine subcutaneously with conspicuous success,[2] while Claude Bernard achieved the same effect in a dog,[3] and began teaching this approach of 'mixed anaesthesia' for operations and in obstetrics.[4] Guibert, following Bernard's lead, noted a bradycardia (54 per min) while using mixed anaesthesia for mastectomy, which resolved 30 min after operation,[5] presumably due to the side-effect of morphine.

The development of regional analgesic techniques has played a vital part in the perfection of postoperative pain control.

Patient controlled analgesia

This was seen as a significant step forward in the relief of suffering, both postoperatively and in other settings. As early as 1960, obstetric patients controlled their own analgesia by screwing a gate clamp on an intravenous pethidine infusion.[6] Sechzer coined the term 'patient controlled analgesia' in 1967, developing a press-button method of delivery of opioids.[7]

In 1971, Keeri-Szanto described the requirements and problems associated with equipment for patient controlled analgesia, observing that since there is enough opiate drug connected to the vein of the patient to produce immediate respiratory arrest, fail-safe methods of control are required in the devices used. In spite of such controls, opiate overdosage continues to occur rarely,[8] due for example to the syringe device being placed high above the patient. This method of analgesia was shown later to reduce postoperative morbidity.[9]

Although the problem of acute postoperative pain was being seriously addressed in Oxford[10] in 1961, a formative report on control of postoperative pain by the Royal College of Anaesthetists and the Royal College of Surgeons of England was produced in 1991, and has encouraged the development of acute pain services throughout the hospitals of the UK.

The management of chronic pain[11]

In 1953 in Liverpool, Sampson Lipton (1922–94)[12] decided to develop a specialized unit, The Centre for Pain Relief, which later became the Pain Research Institute at Walton Hospital. There were major problems with setting up the administration. In the following years, they performed nearly 1000 percutaneous cordotomies. They were the first NHS clinic to use acupuncture. Lipton became medical director of the Pain Research Institute, received the OBE in 1984 and the Pask Certificate of Association of Anaesthetists 1986. He was awarded the MD (Hon) Liverpool 1987. He was a founder member of the International Association for the Study of Pain, the second President of the Intractable Pain Society of Great Britain and Ireland and President of the World Society of Pain Clinicians 1984–91.

The patient with persistent severe pain may require the help of a number of different disciplines. The anaesthetist is likely to be involved in management because of his or her expertise in the use of analgesic drugs and in the performance of nerve blocking techniques. In the UK a number of anaesthetists have been particularly involved in the establishment of multidisciplinary pain clinics. These include Lipton in Liverpool, Swerdlow in the Hope Hospital at Salford,[13] Mark Mehta in Norwich, Lloyd in Oxford and many others. Other prominent pioneer anaesthetists in the field of chronic pain included Bonica in the USA,[14] and Ibsen in Copenhagen. Workers in Mainz have stressed the importance of an interdisciplinary approach.[15]

Examples of some interesting early techniques included hypertonic saline injections into the spinal canal with barbotage.[16] Intrathecal and extradural opiates were used soon after their discovery.[17] Blocks of the autonomic system also rapidly found a place,[18] together with intravenous sympathetic blockade.

References

1. Annotation. *Lancet*, 1863, **1**, 148
2. Annotation. *Med. Times. Lond.*, 1864, **1**, 259
3. Annotation. *Dent. Rev.*, 1864, **NS1**, 203
4. Bernard, C. *Leçons sur les Anaesthésiques et sur l'asphyxie*, Paris, 1871, p.234
5. Guibert L. *C. R. Acad. Sci. Paris*, 1872, **74**, 815
6. Scott, J.S. *Am. J. Obst. Gynecol.*, 1970, **106**, 959–978
7. Sechzer, P.H. *Rev. Argent. Angiology*, 1967, **1**, 9–12; *Anesthesiology*, 1968, **29**, 209–210; *Anesthesiology*, 1990, **72**, 735–736
8. Grover, E.R. and Heath, M.L. *Anaesthesia*, 1994, **47**, 402–404; Notcutt, W.G., Knowles, P. and Kaldas, R. *Br. J. Anaesth.*, 1992, **69**, 95–97; Southern, D.A. and Read, M.S. *Br. Med. J.*, 1994, **309**, 1002
9. Waysylak, T.C., Abbott, F.V.; English, M.J.M. *et al. Can. Anaesth. Soc. J.*, 1990, **37**, 726–731
10. Simpson, B.R.J. and Parkhouse, J. *Br. J. Anaes.*, 1961, **33**, 336–44; Parkhouse, J. *et al. Br. J. Anaes.*, 1961, **33**, 345–353
11. Swerdlow, M. *Anaesthesia*, 1992, **47**, 977–980
12. Obituary. *Br. Med. J.*, 1995, **310**, 1000
13. Swerdlow, M. *Br. J. Clin. Pract.*, 1972, **26**, 403
14. Bonica, J.J. and Black, R.G. In *Relief of Intractable Pain*, edited by M. Swerdlow, Excerpta Medica, Amsterdam, 1974, p.16
15. Gerbershagen, I.I.U., Frey, R., Magin, F., Scholl, N. and Müller-Suur, N. *Br. J. Anaesth.*, 1975, **47**, 526–529
16. Hitchcock, E. and Prandini, M.N. *Lancet*, 1973, **1**, 310–312; Lloyd, J.W., Hughes, J.T. and Davies-Jones, G.A.B. *Lancet*, 1972, **1**, 354–355
17. Behar, M., Magior, F., Olshwang, D. and Davidson, J.T. *Lancet*, 1979, **1**, 527–530
18. Reid, W.J., Watt, J.K. and Gray, T.G. *Br. J. Surg.*, 1970, **57**, 45–50

20
Calendar of interesting and important events in the history of medicine and anaesthesia

500 BC Opium analgesia described by Hippocrates.

150 BC Syringe described by Heron of Alexandria.

100 BC Mandragora analgesia and amnesia described by Dioscorides.

AD 250 Cannabis used for anaesthesia by Hua T'o.

1200 Inhalation of vapour of the soporific sponge described by Nicholas of Salerno.

1516 Curare, South American arrow poison, described by Peter Martyr Angherius.

1518 Foundation of the College of Physicians in London.

1540 Valerius Cordus (1515–44) synthesized sweet oil of vitriol (ether), possibly aided by Theophrastus Bombast von Hohenheim, named Paracelsus (1493–1541).

United Company of Barber Surgeons given Royal Charter by Henry VIII.

1543 Andreas Vesalius (1514–64) of Basel, Louvain and Padua published his revolutionary book on anatomy *De Humani Corporis Fabrica*. As Professor of Surgery and Anatomy at Padua, he replaced moribund mediaeval scholarship by detached scientific observation. He performed intermittent positive pressure ventilation (IPPV) on a pig using a tracheostomy.

Publication of *The Revolutions of the Heavenly Spheres* by Copernicus.

1596 Walter Raleigh describes South American arrow poison.

1628 William Harvey (1578–1657) of London described the circulation of the blood in his book *De Motu Cordis* (Fitzeri, Frankfurt). He was a pupil of Galileo (1564–1642) of Padua and contemporary of Francis Bacon (1561–1626), English philosopher, and of Descartes (1596–1660), French philosopher.

1646 Bartholin described the use of refrigeration anaesthesia by Severeno in *De Novis Usu Medico*.

1662 Robert Boyle (1627–91) enunciated his law of the relationship of the volume and pressure of a gas at a constant temperature.

1665 First intravenous injection of a drug (tincture of opium) into an animal (a dog) by Sir Christopher Wren (1633–1723) and Robert Boyle using a bladder attached to a sharpened quill.

1666 Richard Lower (1631–91) transfused blood from one animal to another.

1667 Robert Hooke (1635–1703), Curator of the Royal Society, performed IPPV on a dog using bellows via a tracheostomy. Denis attempted animal-to-man transfusion.

1707 Sir John Floyer (1649–1734) of Lichfield was the first physician to time the pulse during his clinical examination of patients.

1724 'Anaesthesia' defined in Bailey's *English Dictionary* as 'a defect of sensation'.[1]

1730 August Siegmund Frobenius, a German chemist, living in London, named 'sweet oil of vitriol' ether.

1733 Stephen Hales (1677–1761) inserted tubes into the arteries and veins of animals; the first experiments in direct measurement of blood pressure.[2]

1742 Anders Celsius (1701–44) of Sweden described his system of thermometry, which has displaced the Centigrade scale.

1754 Carbon dioxide ('fixed air') discovered by J. B. von Helmont (1577–1644), Belgian physician, and isolated by Joseph Black (1728–99) in 1757.

1761 Joseph Leopold Auenbrugger (1722–1809) in Vienna described percussion of the chest.

1766 Mesmer described hypnosis.

1768 Wm Heberden (1710–1801), of London, described angina of effort.[3]

1771 Discovery of oxygen by Joseph Priestley (1733–1804) and Carl Wilhelm Scheele (1742–86) of Uppsala, independently.

1772 Priestley discovered nitrous oxide.

1777 Antoine Lavoisier (1743–94) of Paris, scientist and tax collector, named the 'new air' of Priestley 'oxygen' and demolished the phlogiston theory which supposed that only substances containing phlogiston would burn and in so doing would lose their phlogiston.

1785 William Withering (1741–99) described digoxin in *Account of the Foxglove*.

1788 J. A. C. Charles (1746–1823) of France formulated his law of the volume and temperature relationship of a gas at constant pressure.

Chas. Kite of Gravesend first used tracheal tubes in resuscitation of the drowned.

1794 Thomas Beddoes (1760–1808) founded the Pneumatic Institute in Bristol for the treatment of pulmonary tuberculosis and experimented with the therapeutic inhalation of gases and vapours. Humphry Davy (1773–1829) appointed superintendent in 1798.

1796 James Moore compressed nerves to produce local anaesthesia.

1799 Davy suggested analgesic potential of nitrous oxide and named it 'laughing gas'.

1800 Royal College of Surgeons of England given Royal Charter by George III (1738–1820).

1803 Isolation of morphine from opium by Friedrich Wilhelm Adam Seturner (1783–1841), a Paderborn pharmacist. (It was eventually synthesized in 1952.)

1807 Baron Larrey (1766–1842), Napoleon's Surgeon-in-Chief, noticed that amputations were painless when the limbs of wounded soldiers were cold, on the battlefield of Preuss Eylan. The French military surgeons carried out many amputations of frozen limbs. He used triage in evacuation of the wounded.

Seishu Hanaoka (1760–1835) of Hirayama, Japan used a mixture of alkaloids, mainly scopolamine and atropine ('tsusensan') in October 1807 for the first time, to give pain relief to a 60-year-old woman for the removal of a breast cancer.[4]

1811 Charles Bell (1774–1842) of Edinburgh published his *Idea of a New Anatomy of the Brain* in which he differentiated motor nerves and sensory nerves.

1818 Michael Faraday (1779–1867) is said to have discovered the narcotic action of ether vapour. Blundell managed man-to-man transfusion.

1819 Renée Läennec (1781–1826) of Paris invented a stethoscope (*stethas* the chest; *skapeein* to explore).[5] The binaural stethoscope was introduced by Camman in 1855.

1822 François Magendie (1783–1855) of Paris proved in humans that while anterior spinal roots are motor, posterior roots are sensory: 'insensible' and 'sensible' nerves.

1824 Henry Hill Hickman (1800–30) of Ludlow, England carried out operations on animals under carbon dioxide, with freedom from pain, thus establishing the principle of inhalation anaesthesia.

1825 Waterton carried out experiments with curare, using IPPV.

1829 Cloquet used hypnosis for a mastectomy.

1831 Chloroform discovered independently by von Liebig (1830–73) in Darmstadt, Germany, Guthrie (1782–1848) in New York and Soubeiran (1793–1858) in France.

Atropine prepared from *Atropa belladonna*, by Mein, a German pharmacist,[6] and by P. L. Geiger (1785–1836), Professor of Pharmacy of Heidelberg and Hesse.

1832 Thomas Aitchison Latta used intravenous saline in the treatment of circulatory collapse in cholera (not in surgical shock).

1833 Marshall Hall (1790–1857), English physician, introduced the concept of reflex action. Thomas Graham (1805–69), a Scottish chemist, published *On the Law of the Diffusion of Gases*.

1834 Jean-Baptiste Dumas (1800–84) in Paris described chemical composition of, and gave name to, chloroform.

1842 Ether given by W. E. Clarke (1818–78) of Rochester, New York, for dental extraction, and by Crawford W. Long (1815–78) on 30 March in Jefferson, Georgia (the patient, John Venable).[7]

Marie Jean Pierre Flourens (1794–1867), Paris physiologist, first isolated the respiratory centre in the medulla.

1843 Royal Charter given by Queen Victoria (1819–1901) to Royal College of Surgeons of England. Establishment of FRCS (England) diploma. Elliotson described hypnosis for anaesthesia.

1844 Horace Wells (1815–48), a dentist of Hartford, Connecticut, introduced nitrous oxide inhalation to produce anaesthesia during dental extraction. E. R. Smilie used ethereal tincture of opium fumes for anaesthesia in Boston, Mass.

Francis Rynd (1801–61), a surgeon of Dublin, invented the hypodermic trocar.

1846   William T. G. Morton (1819–68), a Boston dentist, successfully demonstrated the anaesthetic properties of ether on 16 October. The patient was Gilbert Abbott (1825–55), a not very robust printer/editor, for a congenital vascular malformation of the floor of the mouth and tongue, and the surgeon J. C. Warren. The patient remained in hospital for 7 weeks.[8] The word 'anaesthesia' was suggested by Oliver Wendell-Holmes (1809–94), Boston academic and writer, for Morton's 'etherization'.

Tooth extracted and ether administered by a dentist, Mr Robinson, in London, 19 December. Dr Francis Boott (1792–1863) was in attendance at 52 Gower Street (now Bonham Carter House, London).[9]

First surgical operation performed in England under ether anaesthesia by Robert Liston (1794–1847), 21 December, when Frederick Churchill (b.1810), a butler, underwent amputation through the thigh. William Squire (1825–99), a medical student, gave the anaesthetic using a glass inhaler at University College Hospital (North London Hospital). Ether also used in Scotland (Dumfries).

1847   Marie Jean Pierre Flourens (1794–1867), Paris physiologist, described anaesthetic properties of chloroform and ethyl chloride vapour in animals.

James Y. Simpson (1811–70) on 8 November introduced chloroform into clinical practice for surgery. He had used diethyl ether earlier that year in Edinburgh to relieve labour pains – the first obstetric anaesthetic. Soon afterwards he used chloroform for the same purpose.

James Robinson published *A Treatise on the Inhalation of the Vapour of Ether.*

John Snow (1813–58), London practitioner, published his book, *On the Inhalation of Ether in Surgical Operations*, the first scientific description of its clinical uses, physical, pharmacological properties, and five stages of narcotism.

Deaths from ether reported from Grantham and Colchester.[10]

1848   Hannah Greener, aged 15, died from chloroform administered by Dr Meggison on 28 January for removal of toenail. Resuscitation was attempted by administering brandy! This was the first recorded death purely related to anaesthesia (at Winlayton, Co. Durham), 11 weeks after the introduction of chloroform into medicine.[11]

Johan Heyfelder (1798–1869) of Erlangen first used ethyl chloride in humans and was the first to use ether in Germany (in 1847).

1849   First anaesthetic death in a London teaching hospital (under chloroform, on 10 October, at St. Thomas's Hospital).[12]

1850 William Gairdner (1824–1907) of Glasgow differentiated between postoperative pneumonia and pulmonary collapse, the latter due to bronchial obstruction.

1853 John Snow (1813–58), London physician and anaesthetist, gave chloroform analgesia on 7 April to Queen Victoria (1819–1901) at the birth of Prince Leopold (1853–81), later Duke of Albany, hence *'chloroform à la reine'*. Sir Charles Locock (1799–1875) was the accoucheur.

Invention of hypodermic syringe and needle by Alexander Wood (1817–74) of Edinburgh.

1855 Friedrich Gaedicke of Germany isolated cocaine from coca plant.

Indirect laryngoscopy described by Manuel Garcia (1805–1906), a Spanish singing teacher working in London.

Foundation of the British Medical Association which developed from Sir Charles Hastings's Worcester Medical and Surgical Society.

1857 Claude Bernard (1813–78), physiologist of Paris, showed that curare acts on the myoneural junction.[13] John Snow, London physician and anaesthetist, gave chloroform analgesia on 14 April to Queen Victoria (1819–1901) at the birth of Princess Beatrice.

1858 Publication of John Snow's book *On Chloroform and Other Anaesthetics*.

General Medical Council established in the UK to supervise medical registration, education and professional conduct.

P. Matthews described electrical anaesthesia, published in the *Medical Times Gazette*, 16 October 1858, p.412.

1859 First examination for the MRCP (London) held.

Charles Darwin (1809–82) published *On The Origin of Species by Means of Natural Selection*.

1860 Albert Niemann (1834–61) purified the alkaloid which Gaedicke had isolated from coca leaves. He named it cocaine.

1861 I. P. Semmelweiss (1818–65) a Hungarian obstetrician, demonstrated in Vienna that puerperal fever is both infectious and contagious.

1862 Thomas Skinner, a Liverpool obstetrician, introduced his domette-covered, wire-framed mask for the administration of volatile anaesthetics, frequently imitated since (e.g. by Curt Schimmelbusch (1860–95), of Berlin, in 1890).

Clover invented his chloroform inhaler.

1863   Gardner Quincy Colton (1817–98) popularized the use of nitrous oxide in dentistry (neglected since Horace Wells's discovery in 1844), by founding the Colton Dental Association.

Louis Pasteur (1822–95) showed that micro-organisms cause fermentation, which led Lister to his discovery of antisepsis in 1865.

1864   Report of Chloroform Committee of Royal Medical and Chirurgical Society, which confirmed chloroform's position as the favoured agent, although ether was shown to be safer.

Johan Nepomuk von Nussbaum (1829–90), surgeon of Munich, gave morphine preoperatively to prolong the action of chloroform.

1867   Professor J. Lister (1827–1912) of Glasgow used carbolic acid to treat the compound fracture of James Greenlees's leg. This was the birth of antiseptic surgery (12 August) in Glasgow.[14] Ferdinand Edelberg Junker (von Laugegg) (1828–1902), Austrian surgeon working in London, described his chloroform insufflation apparatus.

1868   Edmund Andrews (1824–1904), surgeon of Chicago, combined oxygen with nitrous oxide.[15] Thomas Wiltberger Evans (1825–97), American dentist working in Paris, who had learnt about nitrous oxide administration from Colton in 1867, introduced it to London dentists. In the following year, nitrous oxide was supplied in cylinders in compressed form commercially 4 years before US manufacturers put it on the market. Supplies of nitrous oxide may well have been obtainable in London in 1856 from the Medical Pneumatic Appliance Co. (Barth).

C. A. Wunderlich (1815–77) of Leipzig published his work on medical thermometry: *Temperature in Diseases: A Manual of Medical Thermometry* (New Sydenham Society, London), 1868: 'He found fever a disease and left it a symptom' (C. Garrison).

1869   Nasal nitrous oxide inhaler used (independently) by Joseph Thomas Clover (1825–82) and Alfred Coleman (1828–1902), London dentist.

1870   Gustav Simon (1827–1913) of Heidelberg performed the first nephrectomy.

Nitrous oxide cylinders were further developed by S. S. White.

1871   Friedrich Trendelenburg (1844–1924), surgeon from Rostock, Germany, gave anaesthetics via a tracheostomy wound; in 1869 he had used a cuffed tracheostomy tube.[16]

1872   Antisalivary effects of atropine described by R. P. H. Heidenhain (1834–97), Breslau (Wroclaw) physician.

In England, use of ether became much more frequent following the visit of B. Joy Jeffries, an ophthalmic surgeon of Boston, Massachusetts, USA. He advocated the American method of ether administration to British surgeons and anaesthetists, a method involving forcing ether on to the patient who was, if necessary, held down during induction. Previously in Britain, chloroform was used almost exclusively.

Pierre-Cyprien Oré (1828–89) of Bordeaux produced general anaesthesia with intravenous chloral hydrate in animals and two years later applied the method in man.[17]

Clover introduced his nitrous oxide and ether sequence at the British Medical Association Annual Meeting at Norwich.

1874 Forné, French naval surgeon, gave chloral hydrate by mouth to produce sleep before chloroform anaesthesia.

1875 Richard Caton (1842–1926) of Liverpool demonstrated the presence of electric currents in the brain and so was the pioneer of electroencephalography.

1876 Hyperventilation (which produced hypocapnia) with air shown to have analgesic effects by Bonwill.[18]

1877 Joseph Clover introduced his portable regulating ether inhaler.

1880 W. MacEwen (1848–1924), Glasgow surgeon, introduced tracheal intubation by mouth.[19]
Nitrous oxide used for obstetric analgesia.

1881 Stanislaw Klikovich (1853–1910), surgeon of St. Petersburg, used nitrous oxide and oxygen to ease labour pains,[20] a technique later employed by Frederick Hewitt in 1887.

Friedrich Trendelenburg (1844–1924), Professor of Surgery at Rostock, Germany (afterwards at Bonn and Leipzig), introduced the head-down tilt with pelvic elevation, for abdominal surgery.

First successful partial gastrectomy performed by Theodore Billroth (1829–94) at Allgemeine Krankenhaus on 29 January on Therese Heller, in Vienna.[21] First successful gastrojejunostomy performed by A. Woelfler (1850–1917).[22]

1882 Synthesis of cyclopropane by August von Freund (1835–92), Viennese chemist.

Robert Koch (1843–1910), Berlin physician, described the tubercle bacillus.

1884 Koller, Vienna ophthalmologist, demonstrated local analgesic properties of cocaine on the cornea (in a paper read by Joseph Brettauer) (1835–1905) of Trieste, at the Ophthalmological Congress at Heidelberg. W. Stewart Halsted (1852–1922) and Richard John Hall (1856–97), in New York, did the first nerve block with cocaine: the nerve was the mandibular.

Rickman J. Godlee (1849–1925), Lister's nephew and biographer, performed the first operation for the removal of a cerebral tumour.[23]

1885 J. L. Corning (1855–1923), New York neurologist, produced analgesia by the accidental subarachnoid or extradural injection of cocaine in dogs and later humans.

Medical Defence Union founded in London.

1886 Ernst von Bergmann (1836–1907), Berlin surgeon, introduced heat sterilization, the beginning of aseptic surgery.

Corning published the first textbook on local analgesia.

1887 Sir Frederick Hewitt (1857–1916), London anaesthetist, invented the first practical gas and oxygen machine.

1888 First Hyderabad Chloroform Commission.

1889 Second Hyderabad Chloroform Commission. Reports stated that chloroform is never a cardiac depressant and that breathing stops before the heart. This is now known to be untrue. Both Commissions were financed by the Nizam of Hyderabad, Mir Mahbad Ali Khan (1866–1911), who was only 3 years old when he became Nizam.

1890 P. Vera Redard of Geneva introduced the ethyl chloride spray for local analgesia.

W. Stewart Halsted (1852–1922), Professor of Surgery at the Johns Hopkins Hospital, Baltimore, introduced rubber gloves for surgery. Paul Reclus (1847–1914), Paris surgeon, advocated infiltration analgesia with cocaine.

1891 Lumbar puncture demonstrated to be a practical clinical procedure by H. I. Quincke (1842–1922) of Kiel, Germany, and by Essex Wynter (1860–1945), a physician at the Middlesex Hospital in England.

1892 The term 'nerve blocking' introduced by François Frank.[24] Heinrich Braun introduced the term 'conduction anaesthesia'. Karl Ludwig Schleich (1859–1922) of Berlin introduced infiltration analgesia.

1893 London Society of Anaesthetists founded by F. W. Silk of King's College Hospital, London, with Woodhouse Braine as its first president. Other early presidents were G. Hewlett Bailey (in 1896–98) and Dudley W. Buxton (in 1897–98).[25] It became the Section of Anaesthetics of the Royal Society of Medicine in 1908.

1894   Ernest Amory Codman (1869–1940) and Harvey Cushing (1869–1939) in Baltimore advocated use of anaesthetic record charts. Later, 1901, blood-pressure readings, taken with a Riva-Rocci instrument, were added to these charts. (Scipione Riva-Rocci (1863–1937) of Padua.)

1895   X-rays discovered on 8 November by Wilhelm Konrad v. Roentgen (1845–1923) of Würzburg, Nobel prizewinner, 1901 (1st award).

1898   August Bier (1861–1949), surgeon of Kiel, induced first successful clinical spinal analgesia. Theodore Tuffier (1857–1929) of Paris developed and popularized spinal analgesia.

Diamorphine introduced.

Transactions of the Society of Anaesthetists founded in 1893 and published fairly frequently from this date.

1899   Rudolf Matas (1865–1957), New Orleans surgeon, adapted the technique of artificial respiration with bellows (the Fell-O'Dwyer technique) to thoracic surgery.[26]

1900   Karl Landsteiner (1868–1943), of the University of Vienna, later of the Rockefeller Institute, New York City, Nobel prizewinner, 1930, described ABO blood groups.

1901   Extradural caudal injection introduced by Jean-Athanase Sicard (1872–1929), a neurologist of Paris, and Fernand Cathelin (1873–1945), a surgeon of Paris, independently.

First awards of Nobel prizes established by Alfred Bernhard Nobel, Swedish chemist and inventor of dynamite.

Franz Kuhn of Kassel published his work on tracheal intubation.[27]

1902   Heinrich Braun (1862–1934), Leipzig surgeon, added adrenaline to cocaine solution to prolong its effect and retard its absorption.

A. G. Vernon Harcourt (1832–1919), FRS, Reader in Chemistry at Christ Church, Oxford, described his chloroform inhaler in which the concentration of vapour could be measured and its volume regulated, e.g. 2% at temperatures between 16° and 18°C.

E. H. Embley, anaesthetist of Melbourne, Australia described death due to vagal inhibition of the heart during chloroform anaesthesia.[28]

1903 Barbitone (veronal) synthesized by Emil Fischer (1852–1919), Berlin chemist and Nobel prizewinner, 1902, and von Mering (1849–1908) of Munich. This was the first barbiturate.

Willhelm Einthoven (1860–1927) of Leiden, Holland, applied the principles of the string galvanometer to electrocardiographic recording and for this was awarded the Nobel prize for medicine in 1924.[29]

1904 Ernest Fourneau (1872–1949) of Paris synthesized stovaine. Procaine synthesized by Alfred Einhorn (1856–1917), Munich chemist.

1905 The first society of anaesthetists founded in the USA by G. A. F. Erdmann, the Long Island Society of Anesthetists, later (1911) combined with a group from Manhattan to form the New York Society of Anesthetists. In 1935 the organization became national, and in 1936 was named the American Society of Anesthetists Inc. In 1945 the title was changed to the American Society of Anesthesiologists Inc., at the suggestion of Paul Wood (1897–1963), New York anaesthetist, the name 'anesthesiology' having been coined by Seifert in 1902.
Procaine used by Heinrich Braun (1862–1934).

1907 Arthur E. Barker (1850–1916), surgeon, of University College Hospital, London, made use of the curves of the vertebral column in spinal analgesia and introduced hyperbaric solutions of stovaine in 5% glucose. The pioneer of spinal analgesia in Britain.[30]
Foundation of the Royal Society of Medicine in London.
Chevalier Jackson (1865–1958), of Philadelphia, described his work on laryngoscopy.

1908 Massive collapse of the lungs described by Wm Pasteur, English physician (1856–1943).[31]
Louis Ombrédanne (1871–1956), Paris surgeon, described his ether–air inhaler.
Bier described intravenous procaine regional analgesia. J. Goyanes, a Spanish surgeon, described intra-arterial regional anaesthesia.
George Washington Crile (1864–1943), of Cleveland, Ohio, surgeon, described his theory of 'anociassociation'.[32]
The London Society of Anaesthetists became the Section of Anaesthetics of the Royal Society of Medicine.

1909 S. J. Meltzer (1851–1920) and J. Auer (1875–1948), of the Rockefeller Institute, NY used tracheal insufflation anaesthesia in animals.
First Nobel prize awarded to a surgeon, Theodore Kocher of Berne (1841–1907), for his work on the treatment of goitre.
Papaveretum introduced.

1910 C. A. Elsberg (1871–1948), New York surgeon, applied Meltzer and Auer's technique to man (tracheal intubation). Moss introduced clinically practical blood transfusion.

Elmer Ira McKesson (1881–1935) of Toledo, Ohio, anaesthetist and inventor, introduced the first on-demand intermittent-flow gas and oxygen machine, with percentage calibration of the two gases.[33]

Arthur Läwen (1876–1958) of Königsberg showed that extradural analgesia via the sacral route was a useful and practical method of analgesia.

1911 Goodman Levy (1856–1954) proved that chloroform can cause death (from ventricular fibrillation) in light anaesthesia.[34]

A. E. Guedel (1883–1956), working in Indianapolis, reported on the technique of self-administration of nitrous oxide in obstetrics.[35]

Commencement of the National Insurance Act in the UK with its panel of general practitioners.

Robert Kelly of Liverpool (1879–1944) was first to use insufflation tracheal anaesthesia in England.[36]

1912 Walter Meredith Boothby (1880–1953) of Rochester, Minn. and Frederic Jay Cotton (1869–1938), Boston surgeon, introduced a sight feed gas and oxygen flowmeter.

A. Läwen (1876–1958), Königsberg surgeon, used curare to produce relaxation.

J. B. Herrick (1861–1954), Chicago physician, described the features of acute coronary thrombosis.[37]

Francis Hoeffer McMechan (1879–1939) (later the first editor of *Current Researches in Anesthesia and Analgesia*) founded the American Association of Anesthetists.

1913 Danis was first to describe trans-sacral analgesia.

James Tayloe Gwathmey (1865–1944) of New York introduced rectal oil–ether, and in the following year published his classic textbook *Anesthesia*, Appleton, New York.

1914 Albert Hustin of Belgium (1882–1907) was first to use citrate in blood transfusion.

Anesthetic supplements to the *American Journal of Surgery* commenced quarterly publication. This was the first official regularly published literature devoted to the speciality, edited by Francis Hoeffer McMechan (1879–1939), and continued in the USA until 1926.

1915 Use of carbon dioxide absorption in animals by Dennis Jackson of St. Louis, later of Cincinnati.[38]

1916 Sir Francis E. Shipway (1875–1968) of Guy's Hospital, London, introduced his warm ether insufflation apparatus.[39]

1917 Edmund Boyle (1875–1941) of St. Bartholomew's Hospital, and Geoffrey Marshall, London, described their portable nitrous oxide and oxygen machines.

Avertin described by Fritz Eicholtz (1889–1968), pharmacologist, of Heidelberg.

1919 The American Association of Anesthetists founded by James T. Gwathmey (1865–1944) and Frank McMechan (1879–1939).

1920 Guedel's first paper on signs of anaesthesia. These supplanted Snow's signs. Ivan Whiteside Magill (1888–1986) and E. Stanley Rowbotham of London (1890–1979) developed endotracheal anaesthesia.

1921 Extradural lumbar analgesia described by Pagés (1886–1923) of Spain.

1922 *Current Researches in Anesthesia and Analgesia* appeared in August. Founded and edited by Dr F. H. McMechan (1879–1939) and sponsored by the National Anesthetic Research Society in the USA. In 1957 its name was changed to *Anesthesia and Analgesia Current Researches*. It was the first journal to appear regularly in the world exclusively devoted to anaesthesia.

Labat's (1877–1934) *Regional Anesthesia* published.

1923 Carbon dioxide absorption used in man by Ralph Milton Waters.

British Journal of Anaesthesia first published.

1924 Howard Wilcox Haggard (1891–1959) of Yale University published his classic papers on 'The absorption, distribution and elimination of ether'.[40] Intravenous somnifaine was used clinically.

1926 Concept of 'balanced anaesthesia' put forward by J. S. Lundy (1894–1972) of the Mayo Clinic.[41]

Otto Butzengeiger of Wuppertal-Elberfeld, used tribromethyl alcohol (Avertin).[42]

For the first time there was a Section of Anaesthetics at the annual scientific meeting of the British Medical Association.

1927 Ocherblad and Dillon of Kansas City used ephedrine in spinal analgesia to prevent hypotension.

Pernocton used in Germany by R. Bumm. The first barbiturate routinely used for induction of anaesthesia.

1928 Lucas and Henderson in Toronto proved that cyclopropane had anaesthetic properties.

I. W. Magill popularized blind nasal intubation.

1929 Alexander Fleming (1881–1955) of St. Mary's Hospital, London, Nobel prizewinner in 1945, discovered that the mould *Penicillium notatum* secreted an antistaphylococcal substance.[43] This discovery was exploited later for clinical purposes.

1930 Introduction of circle method of carbon dioxide absorption by Brian Sword (1889–1956) of New Haven, Conn.[44]

1931 Achille Mario D. Dogliotti (1897–1966) of Turin reintroduced extradural analgesia in Italy, and four years later founded the Italian Society of Anaesthetists. Foundation of the Liverpool Society of Anaesthetists, the oldest provincial society in England.

1932 Helmut Weese (1897–1954), Scharpff and Rheinoff were the first to use hexobarbitone (Evipan),[45] synthesized by Kropp and Taub.

Christopher Langton Hewer's (1896–1986) *Recent Advances in Anaesthesia* published.

Foundation of the Association of Anaesthetists of Great Britain and Ireland (Figure 20.1); the first President was Henry Featherstone (1894–1976) of Birmingham.

1933 A. Evarts Graham (1883–1957) of St. Louis performed the first successful pneumonectomy for cancer.

Ralph Waters (1883–1979) appointed Professor and Chairman of the new Department of Anesthesia in the University of Wisconsin at Madison: the first such appointment in the USA. (Thomas Drysdale Buchanan had been appointed Clinical Professor of Anesthesiology at the College of Physicians and Surgeons of Columbia, New York, a non-university appointment in 1918.)

Divinyl ether introduced, and used in 1:4 combination with ether as 'VAM' (Vinyl ether Anaesthetic Mixture, May & Baker Ltd).

Polyethylene (polythene) synthesized by R. O. Gibson and E. W. Fawcett in the UK. Manufacture commenced in 1939 by Imperial Chemical Industries.

1934 Ralph Waters and associates from Madison, Wisconsin, reported on the clinical use of cyclopropane where it was first administered on 9 October 1930.

J. S. Lundy, anaesthetist of the Mayo Clinic, popularized thiopentone.

Australian Society of Anaesthetists formed.

Brewer-Luckhardt reflex (laryngospasm caused by stimulation of another part of the body) described.

1935 The first commercial intravenous drip.[46]

An Elberfeld chemist with IG Faben Industrie, Gerhardt Domagk

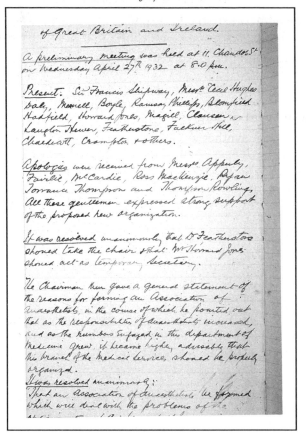

of Great Britain and Ireland.

A preliminary meeting was held at 11 Chandos St on Wednesday April 27th 1932 at 8.0 p.m.

Present: Sir Francis Shipway, Messrs Cecil Hughes Dale, Marwell, Boyle, Ramsay, Phillips, Blomfield Hadfield, Howard Jones, Magill, Clausen, Langton Hewer, Featherstone, Faulkner Hill, Chaldecott, Crompton & others.

Apologies were received from Messrs Apperly, Fairlie, McCardie, Ross Mackenzie, Ryan Torrance Thompson and Thompson Rowling, All these gentlemen expressed strong support of the proposed new organization.

It was resolved unanimously that Dr Featherstone should take the chair & that Mr Howard Jones should act as temporary secretary.

The Chairman then gave a general statement of the reasons for forming an Association of Anaesthetists, in the course of which he pointed out that as the responsibilities of anaesthetists increased, and as the numbers engaged in the department of medicine grew, it became highly advisable that this branch of the medical service should be properly organized.

It was resolved unanimously:
That an Association of Anaesthetists be formed which will deal with the problems of ...

Figure 20.1 **Minutes of the first meeting of the Association of Anaesthetists of Great Britain and Ireland**

(1895–1967),[47] Nobel prizewinner 1939, introduced the first 'sulpha' drug for the control of haemolytic streptococcal infections.

First examination for DA held. H. E. G. Boyle and C. W. Morris were the first examiners.

1936 Successful treatment of puerperal fever with sulphanilamide by C.Leonard Colebrook and Meave Kenny.[48]

McKesson introduced intermittent flow anaesthetic machines.

1937 R. R. Macintosh (1897–1989) appointed Nuffield Professor of Anaesthesia in the University of Oxford, the first chair of anaesthesia in Europe.

American Board of Anesthesiology proposed.

Guedel's *Inhalation Anesthesia* published, describing four stages of unpremedicated ether anaesthesia, and four planes of stage 3.

1938 Positive-pressure respirator used in surgery by Crafoord, surgeon (1899–1984) – the spiropulsator of Paul Frenckner (1986–1967) an otorhinolaryngologist of Stockholm.

American Board of Anesthesiology created, affiliated to the American Board of Surgery.

1939 Pethidine synthesized by Schaumann and Eisleb at Hoechst Farbwerke, Germany.

1940 The journal *Anesthesiology* first published.

Development of controlled breathing by Arthur Guedel (1883–1956) of Indiana, and by Michael Nosworthy (1902–80) of St. Thomas's Hospital, London. In the following 10 years this led the way to the appearance of 'Respiratory Care Units', the forerunners of the modern Intensive Care Units.

Karl Landsteiner (1888–1943) and Alexander Wiener (1906–76) of the Rockefeller Institute, New York City, isolated the Rh factor in blood.

Preparation of an active and concentrated form of penicillin described.[49] Penicillin given on 15 October at Columbia-Presbyterian Hospital, New York to a patient by Dr Aaron Alston.

1941 Trichloroethylene advocated by Langton Hewer and Charles Frederick Hadfield (1875–1965), used for anaesthesia and obstetric analgesia.

American Board of Anesthesiology became independent of the Board of Surgery.

Frank J. Murphy, Detroit anaesthetist, described a lateral opening or eye at the end of a tracheal tube to avoid blocking the right upper lobe bronchus.

1942 Harold Randall Griffith (1894–1985) and G. Enid Johnson of Montreal used curare in anaesthesia.

1943 Macintosh described his curved laryngoscope in Oxford.

The first electronic computer was designed in the USA by Eckert and Mauchley to calculate artillery firing tables (electronic numerical integrator and computer, or ENIAC). It weighed 30 tons and contained 18 000 thermionic valves. Created at the University of Pennsylvania.

W. A. Cobb described the suction catheter-mount connector.

1945 The American Society of Anesthesiologists formed from the American Society of Anesthetists, with the intention of improving education and standards of anaesthesia. It took over the publication of the journal *Anesthesiology*.

1946 Centenary celebrations of anaesthesia.[50]
The journal *Anaesthesia* first published.

1947 First clinical use of lignocaine (Xylocaine) by Torsten Gordh (b.1907) of Stockholm.

1948 Faculty of Anaesthetists established by the Council of the Royal College of Surgeons of England. A. D. Marston (1891–1962), of Guy's Hospital, London, was its first Dean.
First use of hypotensive anaesthesia by H. W. C. Griffiths and John Gillies (1895–1976) in Edinburgh using high spinal analgesia.
Commencement of the two-part Diploma in Anaesthesia (UK) examination.
National Health Insurance started in the UK in July.
Invention of the transistor in the USA.

1949 Penta- and hexamethonium described by W. D. M. Paton and Eleanor Zaimis (1915–83).
Short-acting muscle relaxants described by Daniel Bovet (who was also the first to prepare antihistamines) and used clinically two years later in Italy and Sweden.
Cortisone used at the Mayo Clinic.[51]

1950 Induced hypothermia in cardiac surgery described by Wilfred Gordon Bigelow, surgeon, and his colleagues from Toronto.
Scandinavian Society of Anaesthetists formed. Their first Congress was held in Oslo.

1951 C. W. Suckling of Manchester synthesized halothane.

1952 Faculty of Anaesthetists of the Royal Australasian College of Surgeons founded, and D. Renton was its first Dean. First examination for its fellowship was held in 1956.
Use of IPPV with bag and tracheal tube in Copenhagen polio epidemic.[52]
Pin index system for cylinders introduced.

1953 First examination for Fellowship in Faculty of Anaesthetists of the Royal College of Surgeons of England in London.
First successful open-heart operation performed by John H. Gibbon (1903–74) at Thomas Jefferson Medical School, Philadelphia, using Gibbon extracorporeal bypass apparatus, 6 May.

1954 *Canadian Anaesthetists' Society Journal* first published.

1955 Vibierg Olof Björk and Carl Gunnar Engström, both surgeons, described IPPV for the treatment of postoperative respiratory failure.

World Federation of Societies of Anaesthesiologists formed at the first World Congress of Anaesthesiologists at The Hague. First Congress of the Federation in Scheveningen, Holland.
British Journal of Anaesthesia published monthly.

1956 Michael Johnstone of the Manchester Royal Infirmary used halothane clinically.
American National Standards Committee (Z79) marked implant testing on plastic tracheal tubes.

1957 *Survey of Anesthesiology* and *Acta Anaesthesiologica Scandinavica* first published.
Phenoperidine introduced.

1958 First report of halothane hepatitis.

1959 Faculty of Anaesthetists established by the Royal College of Surgeons in Ireland, with T. Gilmartin as the first dean.
Neurolept analgesia reported by De Castro and Paul Mundeleer.
Lucy Baldwin (1859–1945) obstetric nitrous oxide machine developed.
The analgesic effect of hyperventilatory hypocapnia was discussed by Geddes and Gray.[53]

1960 Fentanyl introduced.

1961 First Coronary Care Units opened for resuscitation after myocardial infarction.
Electrical anaesthesia investigated by Clutton-Brock, Professor of Anaesthesia in Bristol, UK.

1962 First European Congress of Anaesthesiology in Vienna. First Asian-Australasian Congress of Anaesthesiologists held in Manila.
Robertshaw double-lumen tube invented.
Michael Tunstall of Aberdeen, UK used Entonox for the first time.

1963 Committee on Safety of Drugs founded in UK, and became Committee on Safety of Medicines in 1971. Bupivacaine used clinically by L. J. Teluvuo.

1965 Gate theory of pain described by Melzack and Wall.

1966 Ketamine used clinically by Corssen and Domino in the USA.
Enflurane used by Virtue of Denver and his colleagues. Desflurane synthesized.

1967 First heart transplant performed by Christiaan Barnard in South Africa.

The Sanders injector was invented.

1970 Intensive Care Society founded in the UK. Society for Critical Care Medicine founded in the USA.
Central venous cannulas developed for routine use.

1971 First clinical use of isoflurane. First report of sevoflurane.

1973 Long-term central venous catheterization described.[54]
High-frequency jet ventilation developed.
A. I. J. Brain constructed the first laryngeal mask prototype.

1974 Sufentanil introduced.

1976 Alfentanil introduced.

1977 Propofol in Cremophor was introduced.

1981 Association of Anaesthetists set up the first 'sick doctor scheme'.

1982 First Meeting of the European Society of Regional Anaesthesia held in Edinburgh.
First International Symposium on the History of Anaesthesia held in Rotterdam.

1983 Clinical use of laryngeal mask described by A. I. J. Brain.

1984 Propofol in soya bean oil was introduced.

1987 First clinical use of desflurane.

1988 College of Anaesthetists established in London, to supplant the Faculty of Anaesthetists.[55]

1990 *British Journal of Anaesthesia* became the official journal of the College of Anaesthetists.
Sevoflurane used in Japan.

1991 The College of Anaesthetists in London granted its Royal Charter.

References

1. Gillies, J., quoted by Beecher, H.K. *Anesthesiology* 1968, **29**, 1068; see also Miller A.H. *Curr. Res. Anesth. Analg.*, 1928, **7**; 240–247
2. Clark-Kennedy, A.E. *Br. Med. J.*, 1977, **2**, 1656
3. Heberden, W. *Med. Trans. Coll. Phys. Lond.*, 1768, **2**, 59
4. Correspondence. *Anesthesiology* 1970, **33**, 476
5. Bishop, P.J. *J. Roy. Soc. Med.*, 1980, **73**, 448
6. Mein A. *Ann. Pharmacie*, 1833, **6**, 67
7. Young, H. *A Surgeon's Autobiography*, Harcourt Brace, New York, 1940, p.69; see also Hammonds, W.D. (p.256), Papper, E.M. (pp.318–325) and

Stetson, J.B.(pp.400–407), in *The History of Anesthesia, Third International Symposium*, edited by B. R. Fink, L. E. Morris, and C. R. Stephen, Wood Library–Museum of Anesthesiology, Park Ridge, Ill., 1992

8. Eavey, R.D.N. *New Engl. J. Med.*, 1983, **309**, 990
9. Dawkins, R.J. Massey, *Anaesthesia*, 1947, **2**, 51. The letters of Boott to *Lancet*, are reprinted in 'Classical File', *Surv. Anesthesiol.*, 1957, **1**, 65
10. Nunn, R. *Lond. Med. Gaz.*, 1847, **39** (4 n.s.), 414; Annotation, *Lancet*, 1847, **1**, 340
11. Snow, J. *On Chloroform and Other Anaesthetics.* Reprinted in *Br. J. Anaesth.*, 1955, **27**, 501; 'Classical File', *Surv. Anesthesiol.*, 1973, **17**, 381; report of coroner's inquest reprinted in *Surv. Anesthesiol.*, 1959, **3**, 137 and Annotation *Lancet*, 1848, **1**, 161 (reprinted in 'Classical File', *Surv. Anesthesiol.*, 1959, **3**, Feb., 137
12. Wylie, W.D. *Ann. Roy. Coll. Surg.*, 1975, **56**, 171
13. Lee, J.A. *Anaesthesia*, 1978, **33**, 741
14. Lister, J. *Lancet*, 1867, **1**, 326; *ibid.*, **2**, 353
15. 'Classical File', *Surv. Anesthesiol.*, 1963, **7**, 74
16. Trendelenburg, F. *Arch. Klin. Chir.*, 1871, **12**, 112
17. Oré, P-C. *C. R. Acad. Sci. Paris*, 1874, **515**, 651
18. Bonwill, R. *Phil. J. Dent. Science*, 1876, **3**, 37 (reprinted in 'Classical File', *Surv. Anesthesiol.*, 1964, **8**, 348
19. MacEwen, W. *Br. Med. J.*, 1880, **2**, 122
20. Klikovitch, S. *Arch. Gynaek.*, 1881, **18**, 81; Richards, W. *et al. Anaesthesia*, 1976, **31**, 933
21. Billroth, T. *Wien Med. Wochenschr.*, 1881, **31**, 161; Obituary. *Surg. Gynecol. Obst.*, 1979, **148**, 252; Mann, R.J. *Mayo Clin. Proc.*, 1974, **49**, 132
22. Woelfler, A. *Zbl. f. Chirurg.*, 1881, **8**, 705
23. Bennett, H. and Godlee, R.J. *Lancet*, 1884, **2**, 1090
24. Frank, F. *Arch. Physiol. Normal Path.*, 1892, **24**, 562
25. Dinnick, O.P. *Prog. Anaesthesiol.*, Proc. 4th WFSA in London, Amsterdam, Excerpta Medica, Amsterdam, 1970
26. Matas, R. *Ann. Surg.*, 1899, **29**, 426
27. Sweeney, B. *Anaesthesia*, 1985, **40**, 1000
28. Reprinted in 'Classical File', *Surv. Anesthesiol.*, 1965, **9**, 511, 634, from *Br. Med. J.*, 1902, **1**, 817, 885, 951. See also Wilson, G.C.M. *Anaesth. Intensive Care*, 1972, **1**, 9
29. Einthoven, W. *Arch. Ges. Physiol.*, 1903, **99**, 472
30. Lee, J.A. *Anaesthesia*, 1979, **34**, 885
31. Lee, J.A. *Anaesthesia*, 1978, **33**, 362
32. Crile, G.W. *Am. J. Surg.*, 1908, **47**, 864
33. McKesson, E.I. *Surg. Gynecol. Obstet.*, 1911, **13**, 456; see also Waters, R.M. *J. Hist. Med. Allied Sci.*, 1946, **1**, 595
34. Goodman Levy, A. *Chloroform Anaesthesia*, John Bale, Sons and Danielsson, London, 1922
35. Guedel, A. *Indianap. Med. J.*, 1911, **14**, 476
36. Kelly, R. *Br. J. Surg.*, 1911, **1**, 90
37. Herrick, J.B. *J.A.M.A.*, 1912, **59**, 2015

38. Jackson, D. *J. Lab. Clin. Med.*, 1915, **1**, 1
39. Shipway, F.E. *Lancet*, 1916 **1**, 70
40. Haggard, H.W. *J. Biol. Chem.*, 1924, **59,** 737 *et seq.*, reprinted in 'Classical File', *Surv. Anesthesiol.*, 1957, **1**, 629; *Anesth. Anal.*, 1975, **54**, 654
41. Lundy, J.S. *Minn. Med.*, 1926, **9**, 399
42. Butzengeiger, O. *Dtsch. Med. Wochenschr.*, 1927, **53**, 712
43. Fleming, A. *Br. J. Exp. Pathol.*, 1929, **10**, 226
44. Sword, B.C. *Curr. Res. Anesth. Analg.*, 1930, **9**, 198 (reprinted in 'Classical File', *Surv. Anesthesiol.*, 1981, **25**, 65)
45. Weese, H. *et al. Dtsch. Med. Wochenschr.*, 1932, **2**, 1205
46. Marriott, H.L. and Kekwick, A. *Lancet*, 1935, **1**, 977
47. Gerhardt Domagk. *Dtsch. Med. Wochenschr*, 1935, **61**, 250
48. Colebrook, C.L. and Kenny, M. *Lancet*, 1936, **1**, 1279
49. Chain, E.B. *et al. Lancet*, 1940, **2**, 226
50. Bourne, W. *Anesthesiology*, 1948, **9,** 239, 358; *J. Hist. Med. Allied Sci.*, 1946, **1,** no.4, Oct.
51. Hench, P.S. *et al. Proc. Staff Meet. Mayo Clin.*, 1949, **24,** 181
52. Lassen, H.C.A. *Lancet*, 1953, **1,** 37; Ibsen, B. *Proc. R. Soc. Med.*, 1954, **47,** 72
53. Geddes, I.C. and Gray, T.C. *Lancet*, 1959, **2**, 4
54. Broviac, J.W., Cole, J.J. and Scribner, B.H. *Surg. Gyn. Obstet.*, 1973, **136,** 602–606
55. Mushin, W. *Anaesthesia*, 1989, **44,** 291–292

Appendix I The organization of the speciality

Following a joint congress of anaesthetists in London in 1951 of which Sir Ivan Magill was President, and a similar meeting in Paris the same year, it was decided to form a Federation of Societies of Anaesthesiologists and the first Congress of the new body was held in Scheveningen in Holland in 1955. Other similar congresses have been held in Toronto (1960), Sao Paulo (1964), London (1968), Kyoto (1972), Mexico City (1976), Hamburg (1980), Manila (1984), Washington (1988), The Hague (1992) and Sydney (1996). (See also van Lieburg, M.J. In *Anaesthesia: Essays on its History*, edited by J. Rupreht *et al.*, Springer-Verlag: Berlin, 1985, p.307; Organe, G. *ibid.*, p.309; Howat, D.D.C. *ibid.*, p.314; Secher, O. *ibid.*, p.321; Griffith, I I.R. *Anesth. Analg. Curr. Res.*, 1963, **42**, 389; Zorab, J. *Anaesthesia*, 1976, **31**, 285; Boulton, T.B. *Anaesthesia*, 1976, **31**, 1103.)

Among training courses arranged by the World Health Organisation were those of the Anaesthesiology Centre in Copenhagen (1950–73) and in Manila (under the guidance of Professor Quintin Gomez).

Organization of anaesthesia in Britain

See also Dinnick, O.P. *Proc. 4th World Cong. Anaesth.*, London, 1968, p.181.

The Society of Anaesthetists was founded in 1893 by J.F.W.M. Silk (1878–1943) of King's College Hospital, and 40 anaesthetists joined it. First President was Woodhouse Braine (1837–1907) of Charing Cross Hospital, with Silk as Honorary Secretary and Dudley W. Buxton (1855–1931), of University College Hospital, as Treasurer. Published its first volume of *Transactions* in 1898. In 1908 it was incorporated as the Section of Anaesthetics of the new Royal Society of Medicine. It was the first society of anaesthetists in the world which had as its object the discussion of problems of anaesthesia and the advancement of the science and art of the subject. The Scottish Society of Anaesthetists dates from 1914.

The Association of Anaesthetists of Great Britain and Ireland was founded in 1932 to perform functions which could not be performed by the Section of Anaesthetics of the Royal Society of Medicine. These were (and remain): to promote the development and study of anaesthetics and their administration, and the recognition of the administration of anaesthetics as a specialized branch of medicine; to co-ordinate the efforts and activities of anaesthetists; to represent anaesthetists and to promote their interests; to promote the establishment of diplomas and degrees in anaesthesia; to encourage and promote co-operation and friendship between anaesthetists; and finally to do all such lawful things as may be incidental or conducive to the attainment of such objects. The first President was Henry Featherstone (1894–1967) of Birmingham, with W. Howard Jones of Charing Cross Hospital as Secretary and Z. Mennell (1876–1959) of St. Thomas's Hospital, London as Treasurer. At this time there were only 50 specialist anaesthetists in the whole of the UK.

See Hunter, A.R. *Anaesthesia*, 1983, **38**, 1214; Helliwell, P.J. *Anaesthesia*, 1982, **37**, 394, 913; Boulton, T.B. In *A History of Anaesthesia*, edited by R. S. Atkinson and T. B. Boulton, Royal Society of Medicine, London, 1989. For a description of the Arms of the Association, see Boulton, T.B. *Anaesthesia*, 1974, **29**, 627

The Faculty of Anaesthetists of the Royal College of Surgeons of England was created in 1948 at the request of the Association of Anaesthetists. A.D. Marston (1891–1962) of Guy's Hospital was the first Dean. See Atkinson, R.S. In *A History of Anaesthesia*, edited by R. S. Atkinson and T. B. Boulton, Royal Society of Medicine, London, 1989.

The Fellowship (FFARCS, then FCAnaes, and now FRCA) was proposed in 1946 and the first examinations held in 1953. The diplomas were awarded from 1954. The College of Anaesthetists was created in 1989 when a new charter allowed the Faculty of Anaesthetists to evolve to collegiate status. It became the Royal College of Anaesthetists in 1991. The Faculty of Anaesthetists of the Royal College of Surgeons in Ireland was founded in 1959, the first examination for its fellowship taking place in 1961.

Appendix II Early publications on anaesthesia

1824 Henry Hill Hickman wrote a private letter and later an open letter to T.A. Knight on the subject of *Suspended Animation*, giving details of his experiments on dogs and mice. He used carbonic acid gas to render them insensible during the carrying out of surgical procedures with recovery (reproduced in Faulconer, A. and Keys, T.E. *Foundations of Anesthesiology*, Vol. 1, Thomas, Springfield, Ill., 1965).

1846 Bigelow, H.J. Insensibility during surgical operations produced by inhalation. *Boston Medical and Surgical Journal*, **35,** 309–317 (18 November): a paper read on 9 November to the Boston Society of Medical Improvement.

1847 Morton, W.T.G. *Remarks on the Proper Mode of Administering Sulphuric Ether by Inhalation*, 44pp. Printed by Dutton and Wentworth, Boston.

The above are all reproduced in Faulconer and Keys' book (see above).

1846 et seq. Keys, T.E. *The History of Surgical Anesthesia.*, Dover Publications, New York, 1963, pp.183–189, lists early tracts on ether by Morton and Warren.

1847 Wells, H. *A History of the Discovery of the Application of Nitrous Oxide Gas, Ether and Other Vapours, to Surgical Operations*, J. G. Wells, Hartford, Conn.

1847 Robinson, J. *A Treatise on the Inhalation of the Vapour of Ether*, 1st edn, Webster, London. Facsimile edition, with an introductory essay by Richard H. Ellis, Baillière Tindall, Eastbourne, 1983.

1847 Snow, J. *On the Inhalation of the Vapour of Ether in Surgical Operations: Containing a Description of the Various Stages of Etherization and a Statement of the Result of Nearly Eighty Operations in which Ether has been Employed in St. George's and University College Hospitals*, John Churchill, Princes Street, Soho, London.

1847 Heyfelder, J.F. *Die Versuche mit dem Schwefelather und die daraus gewonnenen Resultate in der Chirurgischen Klinik zu Erlangen,* Heyder, Erlangen.

1848 Heyfelder, J.F. *Die Versuche mit dem Schwefelather, Salzather und Chloroform und die daraus gewonnenen Resultate in der chirurgischen Klinik zu Erlangen,* Heyder, Erlangen.

1848 Warren, J.C. *Etherization; With Surgical Remarks,* Ticknor, Boston. Extracts reproduced in Faulconer and Keys (see above).

1848 Anaesthetic agents. *Transactions of the American Medical Associaton* (Instituted 1847), Vol 1.

1849 Long, C.W. An account of the first use of sulphuric ether by inhalation as an anaesthetic in surgical operations. *Southern Medical and Surgical Journal,* **5,** 705–713. Reproduced in Faulconer and Keys (see above).

1858 Snow, J. *On Chloroform and Other Anaesthetics; Their Action and Administration,* edited by B. W. Richardson, John Churchill, New Burlington Street, London.

1880 Morton, W.J. *The Invention of Anaesthetic Inhalation; or, 'Discovery of Anaesthesia',* Appleton, New York.

1881 Lyman, H.M. *Artificial Anaesthesia and Anaesthetics,* Wood, New York.

1884 Koller, C. Vorlaufige Mittheilung uber locale Anasthesirung am Auge. Bericht 16, Versamml d Ophthalmologischen Gesselsch, Heidelb. In *Klinische Monatsblätter für Augenheilkunde,* **22,** Beilageheft, pp.60–63.

1886 Corning, J.L. *Local Anaesthesia in General Medicine and Surgery,* Appleton, New York.

1888 Buxton, D.W. *Anaesthetics: Their Uses and Administration,* H. K. Lewis, London.

1893 Hewitt, F.W. *Anaesthetics and their Administration,* Griffin, London.

For a list of some of the earliest books dealing with anaesthesia, see Secher, O. *Anaesthesia,* 1985, **40,** 385.

Appendix III Books on the history of anaesthesia

Journal of the History of Medicine and Allied Sciences, Anesthesia Centennial Number, Schuman, New York, Oct. 1946

Duncum, B.M. *The Development of Inhalation Anaesthesia – With Special Reference to the Years 1846–1900*, Oxford University Press, London, 1947

Bryce-Smith, R., Mitchell, J.V. and Parkhouse, J. *The Nuffield Department of Anaesthetics, 1937–62*, Oxford University Press, Oxford, 1963

Keys, T.E. *The History of Surgical Anesthesia*, Schuman, New York, 1945. Revised and enlarged version as Dover edition, New York, 1963

Bryn Thomas, K. *Curare – Its History and Usage*, Pitman, London, 1964

Faulconer, A and Keys, T.E. *Foundations of Anesthesiology*, Thomas, Springfield, Ill. (two volumes), 1965

Armstrong Davison, M.H. *The Evolution of Anaesthesia*, John Sherratt, Altrincham, UK, 1965

Bryn Thomas, K. *The Development of Anaesthetic Apparatus*, Blackwell, Oxford, 1975

Smith, W.D.A. *Under the Influence – A History of Nitrous Oxide and Oxygen Anaesthesia*, Macmillan, London, 1982

Sykes, W.D. *Essays on the First 100 Years of Anaesthesia*, Vols 1 and 2, 1961–62, Churchill Livingstone, London and Edinburgh, 1982

Ellis, R.H. (ed.) *Essays on the First 100 Years of Anaesthesia*, Vol. 3, Churchill Livingstone, London and Edinburgh, 1982

Secher, O. *Bibliography on the History of Anaesthesia*, Rigshospitalet, Copenhagen, 1984

Rupreht, J. *et al.* (eds). *Anaesthesia: Essays on its History*, Springer-Verlag, Berlin, 1985

Beinart, J. *A History of The Nuffield Department of Anaesthetics, Oxford, 1937–87*, Oxford Medical Publications, Oxford, 1987

Wilson, G.C. *Fifty Years, History of the Australian Society 1934–1984*, Australian Society of Anaesthetists, Edgecliff, NSW, 1987

Wilson, G.C. (ed.) Thirlwell-Jones, J. *One Grand Chain, The History of Anaesthesia in Australia 1846–1962*, Vol. 1, 1846–1934, Australian and New Zealand College of Anaesthetists, Melbourne, 1955

Proceedings of World Congresses on the History of Anaesthesia

Atkinson, R.S. and Boulton, T.B. (eds). *A History of Anaesthesia*, Royal Society of Medicine, London, 1989

Fink, B.R., Morris, L.E. and Stephen, C.R. (eds. *The History of Anaesthesia: Proceedings of 3rd International Symposium*, Wood Library-Museum, Park Ridge, Ill., 1992

Index